CAUSE AND PREVENTION OF THE DEATH OF HEALTH CARE

CAUSE AND PREVENTION OF THE DEATH OF HEALTH CARE

Len Dartt

iUniverse, Inc.
New York Lincoln Shanghai

CAUSE AND PREVENTION OF THE DEATH OF HEALTH CARE

iUniverse books may be ordered through booksellers or by contacting:

iUniverse
2021 Pine Lake Road, Suite 100
Lincoln, NE 68512
www.iuniverse.com
1-800-Authors (1-800-288-4677)

Because of the dynamic nature of the Internet, any Web addresses or links contained in this book may have changed since publication and may no longer be valid.

The information, ideas, and suggestions in this book are not intended as a substitute for professional medical advice. Before following any suggestions contained in this book, you should consult your personal physician. Neither the author nor the publisher shall be liable or responsible for any loss or damage allegedly arising as a consequence of your use or application of any information or suggestions in this book.

ISBN: 978-0-595-47704-3 (pbk)
ISBN: 978-0-595-91967-3 (ebk)

Printed in the United States of America

Contents

INTRODUCTION

This writer has properly addressed the cause and prevention of the death of health care by properly addressing the cause and prevention of medical problems, period.

All of the talk about universal health care is meaningless, since if the trend continues in health care; there will be no health care universal or otherwise. One look at New England's loss of health care says it all. The article in the media was titled "New Englanders on the Death of Their Health Care". The article was authored by Neal Pierce, syndicated columnist, Washington Post, and Curtis Johnson, public policy analyst. The key points in the article were that making New England healthier means thinking about medicine in a whole new way. New England has more of its work force than any other part of the United States engaged in health care, with more treatments, yet New England residents are not healthier than other parts of the US.. The New England states are not free of spiraling medicare costs. More spending and more treatment are not making New Englander's healthier. Also, despite the fact that New Englander's eat a little less and exercise a little more than other parts of the US they are not healthier. If they require hospital treatment some of the best health care professionals are located in New England. Despite the above, New England is plagued with soaring medical costs, with mediocre health results. Not mentioned in the article but very significant is the fact that New England has the highest rates in the nation of breast cancer and asthma. Massachusetts has one of the highest rates, nationwide, for chronic illnesses. This writer addresses the cause and prevention of the death of health care, in New England, including the cause and prevention of breast cancer, asthma, and chronic illnesses, in the chapter on the Cause and Prevention of Medical Problems.

Also, the Institute of Medicine reported that the American health system is failing. They reported that "health care today harms too frequently and fails to deliver its potential benefits". Along with this report I believe the statement in the New York Times in an article on medical problems summed up the seriousness of the problems. The article said, "There are plenty of medical problems out there but why solve them if there is no money in it".

Within the various chapters, in this book, this writer has provided documented data on the factors leading up to the death of health care. Since I found that the medical scientific establishment and associated foundations did not properly understand and/or properly address these factors it means that the reader, their family, and friends, must attempt to properly address these factors. Within these same chapters I have provided documented data that not only will allow the reader to properly address their health problems, but that the end result will be the prevention of the death of health care.

The reader's attempt to help themselves to a healthier life will not be easy as a result of the barriers set up by the medical establishment as evident in the chapter on Health Care Terrorism.

Ironically, for the reader to be successful in improving their health and preventing the death of health care it will not take more money. If the reader properly addresses the cause and prevention of medical problems, as outlined in the chapter on the cause and prevention of medical problems, it will mean fewer trips to the doctor and/or the hospital and less medications. Also, if the reader properly addresses the cause and prevention of adverse reactions to medications, as outlined in the chapter on the cause and prevention of adverse reactions to drugs, it will not only mean less drugs overall, but the elimination of drugs to treat the adverse reaction to drugs.

Above all, if the reader is successful in the above it may be possible for the reader to duplicate the healthy life of this writer. At the present time, at the age of 77, I am able to maintain a constant weight of 190lbs. on a 6 foot frame. My vital signs are pulse 68, with average 60-100, blood pressure, systolic 112, with average 140 or less, and diastolic 85, with average 85 or less. I require no medications, not even an aspirin. I have no chronic medical problems. I have no connective tissue medical problems despite having played football, hockey, and baseball in high school and football and hockey in college. Also, despite at one time having experienced every possible adverse auto immune reaction I now do not experience any adverse auto immune reactions. I provide some of the reasons for this healthy condition in the chapters on diet, body processes, ingested pollutants, and the prevention of medical problems.

I felt that I required assistance from members of the medical establishment in presenting my findings. I needed their help in evaluating my documented data, and then to use their prestige to present my medical findings to the Public. I felt that the public would be more inclined to believe my findings if they came from a doctor at Harvard Medical. Unfortunately, my attempts to contact them were met with either deadly silence, or I lost your file, and/or I am sorry I am out of the office.

There are two failed contacts that stand out above all the others. These two contacts involved the body's auto immune process. I felt that these two contacts were important since the body's adverse auto immune response is responsible for the majority of all chronic medical problems. When the American Auto Immune Related Disease Association designated the month of May 2007 as autoimmune disease awareness month I E mailed the President of the association and offered to present my findings on the cause and prevention of some autoimmune diseases. The response was nothing but deadly silence. As a result, I made contact with a doctor who was the Director, Autoimmune Research, at a leading University. I E mailed him a copy of my offer to the President and asked him if he could help me to make contact with her. He E mailed me back saying "I am afraid that I cannot help with this issue"." Sorry". As a result of his reply I offered to provide him with documented data on the cause and prevention of some auto immune diseases. His response was nothing but deadly silence.

I was hoping that by providing my many contacts, among the medical establishment, with a copy of this INTRODUCTION, prior to the publishing my book, that it would give them a chance to reconsider their responses of nothing but deadly silence. However, their reactions were nothing but deadly silence.

I believe that it is fair on the part of the reader to speculate on how this writer, began acquiring data on the various medical problems leading up to the pending death of health care. There were two primary events that took place that prompted me to pursue the cause and prevention of the death of health care. In the first event I was taking care of a two year old girl while the father worked and the Mother was having a baby. On this particular day I had the two year old out to the play ground, with her only concern being when she was going to have her lunch and her nap. When her father came home that evening he informed me that he was taking the 2 year old to the pediatrician. I thought to myself it must be for a check up. So, imagine my surprise when upon arriving home from the doctor the father handed me a prescription for 500mg of amoxicillin and asked me if I would get the prescription filled the next day and get her started on it. I raised my concerns to the pharmacist about the large dosage of this drug but I received no reaction. I did not give the two year old any medication and when the father came home I indicated that in my opinion 500mg. was too high a dosage for his daughter. I also indicated that I had severe ear aches as a child and the pain is at times unbearable. I pointed out to him that his daughter not only had no pain, but showed no discomfort. Fortunately, he accepted my advice and did not give his daughter the medication. I later found out that amoxicillin is not to be given to 2 year olds or younger. I also found out that for children over 2 years old the maximum dosage is only 45mg.. In retrospect, I found that the two year old did not have a true ear infection but an inflamed inner ear canal that looks like an ear infection, caused by an adverse autoimmune reaction. Apparently the pediatrician upon finding the severely inflamed inner ear canal was afraid it might lead to meningitis and prescribed the maximum dosage of 500mg. However, any overdose and/or misapplication of amoxicillin may lead to a hearing loss as a former President and a former Miss America will attest to. The next event was when I developed a severely swollen face. I went to an allergy doctor thinking it was an allergy. He indicated that it wasn't an allergy but did not offer any advice as to where I should go to seek help. I then went to my personal care doctor who did not know the cause of my swollen face but offered to medicate. I then went to the emergency room at a medical center in Massachusetts. A women doctor took one look at me and indicated that she thought I had a rare disorder and sent me up to the disorder doctor at the medical center. He correctly diagnosed my medical problem as swollen saliva glands, not a swollen face, and this was a reaction to the rare disorder Sjogren Syndrome. He indicated that the medical establishment did not know what causes Sjogren Syndrome and/or how to treat it. I discovered that my Sjogren Syndrome was caused by ingesting excessive amounts of whey, in margarine, that triggered my body's adverse auto immune process. It just so happened that I had a lot of left over vegetables that had been around for awhile and had to be eaten. I tried to provide my findings to the President of the medical center and the disorder doctor but they would not talk with me.

While the above events were all personal some non personal events prompted my concerns about the pending death of health care. The actions of, at the time the most powerful man in the free world stood out. The first action on his part was his firing of his predecessor's Doctor because he would not give him an allergy shot. The Doctor would not give him the allergy shot because he had no information on his medical history. His next actions took place when he attempted to assure the American public that he was healthy. He took a physical and reported that he checked out ok, but this time of the year, it was during the holiday season, he always had problems with his allergies to the greeneries. He also reported that he was allergic to the cat but he put the cat out at night. A Doctor H., at John Hopkins, and this writer made contact with him but received no response. We both informed him that no one has an allergic reaction to dead greeneries and that putting the cat out at night doesn't solve the problem since the adverse reaction is caused by the protein in the cat dander that is left wherever the cat travels. Most important, the media never reported on this mans incorrect statements. Here it is the most powerful man in the free world, President Clinton, and he is attempting to properly address the American Public's medical problems when he can't properly address his own medical problems.

As a result of my findings on the above medical problems, which led to my findings on other medical problems, it served, in part, as the basis for the need to inform the Public of the pending death of health care, not just in New England, but worldwide.

Finally, it is this writer's intention to donate every single penny received from the sale of this book to research, not on the cure and treatment of breast cancer, but for research on the cause and prevention of breast cancer. Unfortunately, I have a big problem and that is finding anyone who is researching the cause and prevention of breast cancer. I contacted several breast cancer foundations and offered to donate a large sum of money if they would provide me with the name and/or names of anyone researching the cause and prevention of breast cancer. They could not provide me with a single name. Also, the National Institute of Health has awarded 714 research grants on breast cancer, with only one on the cause and prevention of breast cancer. That grant was insignificant since it involved genetics which is an ongoing factor in most medical research.

FACTS AND STATS ON THE DEATH OF HEALTH CARE

Background

The United States ranks 37th in the world in quality of health care. The medical scientific establishment doesn't know what to do about the costly asthma and diabetic epidemic and the obesity epidemic in the United States. The top causes of deaths for those under 80 years old are cancer 400,592, heart 328,037, injuries 87,125, lungs 70,786, strokes 64,282, diabetes 46,946, influenza, 21,607, and kidneys, 20,160. Drawing on the plight of New Englanders on the death of their health care as to quality and finances two Harvard Medical and Public Health School doctors summed up the plight of health care not only in New England but world wide. Doctor B was quoted "consistently there's so much confusion, waste and arrogance in America's health-care system that the only way to save it is to blow it up first". Doctor A was quoted "the system is failing patients-its consumers". "The driving force has become financial returns for medical professionals and companies that make their living off drugs and treatment". Finally, the statement by CEO E of NEHI, ties in with one of this writer's main themes on the cause of the death of health care. She said or words to the effect that upwards of all health care dollars go to expensive diagnosis, treatment, and surgical procedures-not prevention and public health. Compounding the above is the fact that Americans spend 31% of medical costs on administrative costs. As a result of a serious shortage of doctors in key specialties, including anesthesiology, cardiology, and gastroenterology, patients have reported waiting for care. Patients report waiting for health care because of a shortage of doctors. Physician groups say low reimbursement rates and high malpractice premiums are helping to drive physicians into more lucrative jobs. Health illiteracy is a serious problem in the US.. About one half of all adults, in the US., have difficulty understanding, and using information about their health (Michael Woods Medical Journal). 70% of all Americans don't understand their medical diagnosis.

Medical problems

Infectious diseases have increased by 58% over the last ten years. 35% of the population suffers from chronic fatigue and/or chronic insomnia. Leading causes of deaths per 100,000 people in the US., over 65, are 218 pneumonia & influenza, 226 chronic respiratory ailments, and 1,085 cancers. 49% of all Americans lay claim to the fact that they have chronic medical problems and consume 75% of all health care costs. About 15% of all Americans, under the age of 21, have chronic medical problems that they will carry with them into adulthood. The asthma rates are twice that of the 1980's. 53% of all Americans claim they suffer from chronic pain. By the year 2020 there will be 157 million Americans with chronic illnesses. In 2004 7% of American children & adolescents had chronic health conditions that limited them, in 1960 it was only 1.8%. There are 16 cancer deaths for every 1 HIV. death. Of the approximate 185,000 Americans diagnosed with brain cancers most of them will die within 5 to 6 months. Middle age Americans have about a 90% chance of developing high blood pressure. 11 million Americans suffer from silent strokes (since there are no obvious symptoms), while 750,000 suffer strokes, with 450,000 disabilities. 56% of all mothers that take time off from work do so because of, so called, ear infection in children. Every 34 seconds an American dies of heart disease that costs the US. at least 110 billion per year.3.3 million children world wide die of birth defects. (**March of Dime Report**). One in ten women ages 45 to 64 have some form of heart disease, and by the age of 65 the rate is one in every four women.

Middle aged whites are healthier in England. Americans have higher rates of diabetes, heart diseases, strokes, lung disease, and cancer than the English. The richer American health status resembled the health status of the low income English.

The Institute of Medicine reported in 1999 that up to about 98,000 deaths are caused, annually, by medical errors and that they are on the increase. The media reported that birth defects and deaths have doubled over the last five years.

Drug problems

65% of all drugs are prescribed off label (not for the medical problem that was FDA approved). 50% of all Americans don't take their drugs correctly. Americans spend about 142 billion per year on prescription drugs and spend about 177 billion per year to correct the medical problems caused by these medications. Most medication dosages are too high. 50 million Americans from 6 years to 70 years old take blood pressure drugs with only 27.4 million controlling the blood pressure. About 12% of the elderly use about 32%of all drugs prescribed. One out of ever five new drugs has a serious adverse reaction. It is estimated that only 10% of all adverse drug reactions are reported. Drug prices in the US. are 81% higher than 7 other countries. More than 40% of the population is taking at least one prescription drug and one person in every six persons takes three or more drugs. 15.1 million people that are abusing prescriptions drugs exceed the combined number of people abusing cocaine, hallucinogens, inhalants, and heroin. Out of those 15.1 million people 2.3 million are teenagers. About 17 million people are given the wrong drug every year. 20% of all people hospitalized are hospitalized as a result of an adverse reaction to a drug. On 09-10-07 the media reported that adverse drug events doubled from 1998 to 2005.

Pollution problems

While there are many pollutants that may trigger the body's autoimmune process, that in turn may affect a persons health, there are a few that stand out. Fungus, carbon monoxide, and carbon dioxide are all pollutants that one can't smell, feel, and/or see. In addition to these three, the other key pollutants are preservatives and colorants in food, drink, and/or drugs.

The average American carries about five lbs. of undigested, putrefied, red meat, in their gut. Americans consume about 112 kilos per capita of red meat which is nearly 250 lbs. more than any other nation (Germany 89 & Britain 71). Per year about 140,000 people die on the US. highways, while 400,000 die from smoke related problems. At one Harlem hospital it was found that 62% of all newborns had adverse reactions associated with the exposure to passive smoking. Carbon dioxide pollution has increased at an alarming rate. The risk of heart attacks increases by 62% on days of poor air quality. Seafood is the biggest cause of food poisoning with eggs taking second place.

The average person I believe appreciates the importance of not ingesting any bacteria and/or viruses. Also, they appreciate that if they suddenly start sneezing and their nose starts running that they have ingested a pollutant that caused them to have an allergic reaction. However, the average person I believe does not appreciate the fact that some people may ingest peanuts in peanut butter and have an adverse autoimmune reaction to the peanuts resulting in toxic shock and death. Even the not so average person at the time, the most powerful man in the free world, former President Clinton, did not appreciate the seriousness of some ingested pollutants. The basic diet drug that he was taking was removed from the market because of deaths among its users.

FINANCIAL CRISIS LEADING TO THE DEATH OF HEALTH CARE

Federal Reserve chairman Ben Bernanke said the US. government may face a fiscal crisis in the coming decades if it fails to deal with the rising costs of medical benefits for the aging population. If under the circumstances, early and meaningful action is not taken, the US. economy could be seriously weakened, with future generations bearing much of the cost. While official forecasts may show a stable or a narrower budget deficit over the next few years it may just be the calm before the storm. The Medicare deficit will go from 0.5% of GDP. in 2003 to, 10% of GDP by 2030. This will be the largest deficit ever run up by the US. in the past 50 years. Bernanke said that the economic growth spurring revenue today won't resolve the budget's long term challenge, rising debt, which would require increased spending on interest payments. Thus, a vicious cycle may develop in which large deficits would lead to rapid growth in debt and interest payments, which in turn will add to subsequent deficits. Compounding the above is the fact that there will be less members of the younger generation to support the seniors' medical financial problems. If the trend continues, involving the major increases in chronic medical problems, not only will there be fewer members of the younger generation to support the seniors, the younger generation will need financial assistance themselves.

Scripps Howard News Service reported that Medicare is facing Armageddon. Medicare faces significantly greater fiscal challenges. The Medicare hospital insurance trust fund, that pays hospital benefits, already is operating in the red and is projected to run dry by 2020. The impact on the consumers could be substantial; possibly resulting in higher payroll taxes, additional out-of-pocket expenses, or cuts in services offered by the national health care program for senior citizens and others. The department of health and human services reports that 41.7 million people are currently covered under Medicare. Those 41.7 million will wind up costing the program, not counting the drug benefits; a projected $13 trillion. The average monthly premium for drug coverage is now expected to be $37.37 which is an increase of $2.37 over the projection offered in 2003. It was reported that 10% of US. households are taking care of aged relatives amounting to 34 million individuals over 55. They are spending on the average about $5500 which is more that they spend on their own health care

The Associated Press reported that an obesity pandemic threatens to over whelm the health care systems around the globe with illnesses such as diabetes and heart disease. It reported that the cost of treating obesity related health problems was immeasurable on a global scale, but the group estimated it at billions of dollars a year in countries such as Australia, Britain and the United States. Among the most serious problems is the skyrocketing rate of obesity among children which makes them much more prone to chronic diseases as they grow older.

I believe I have solved the obesity pandemic problem by providing data on the cause and prevention of **World wide obesity** in my chapter on the cause and prevention of medical problems.

HEALTH CARE TERRORISM

Keep in mind that the suppression of dissent by world terrorism is as a result of the threat of death to the dissenter. The suppression of dissent on the part of health care terrorism is out of fear of the powerful AMA. and Drug Industry. The two largest contributors to Congress are the AMA. and the Drug Industry, with 14 million and 58 million respectively. One has to ask what is the reason for these large donations to Congress if is not for the suppression of dissent. Some people might think that my experience in attempting to contact Congressman Waxman, of California, might be a prime example of Congress attempting to control dissent. Through the Swedish Consultant I received from the Swedish Sjogren Foundation via E mail, hey://www.sjogrens.com/news.htm, a news letter published by Waxman, titled News and Events. The newsletter called for supporting a house bill, by Waxman, to establish an office of autoimmune disease at the National Institute of Health. The goal was to coordinate autoimmune research among the institutes at the NIH. Also, in the article, it said that the government affairs committee, working with Waxman's, office were instrumental in getting Sjogren Syndrome included in a list of autoimmune diseases mentioned in the bill. Despite several attempts to contact Waxman he would not respond. If he had contacted me I would have informed him that I was correctly diagnosed with Sjogren Syndrome, found the cause, which was the cause of many other autoimmune diseases, and no longer suffer from this disease. I found that the NIH. awarded 51 million in contracts to research autoimmune diseases.

For some examples of the suppression of dissent on the part of health care terrorism please review the following: Based on prior fact finding, my attention was drawn to an article in the media that indicated that the medical profession was alarmed at the high rates of ear infections among children. I attempted to make contact with the reporter, and the editor of the newspaper that printed the article. Despite physically delivering my documented data to the paper I was met with nothing but deadly silence from them. To me it was obvious that they were in fear of alienated the AMA. and/or the Drug Industry. In the documented data that I left off at the newspaper I indicated that I made contact with a leading manufacture of amoxicillin. I informed the product manager about the article in the paper on ear infections and indicated that the so called ear infections were not a true ear infection, but inflamed ears that looked like an ear infection caused by an adverse autoimmune reaction. I further indicated that Amoxicillin, that was once know as the golden medication for ear infections, is now only 30% effective, since it is not being used for a true ear infection. Since this type of product accounts for 900 billion a year in sales the only response he could think of was "you aren't going to alarm the Public are you"? About two years later the media reported that this same reporter, responsible for the media article on the alleged ear infections, died of a drug overdose at a medical center. Based on documented data that I had acquired, I contacted the Director of Public Relations, at the medical center, and indicated to her that I had information on the death of this reporter, that it was not a true overdose. She indicated to me that I should wait awhile until things calm down and the medical center would invite me over so that I may be able to present my data. Immediately, after my contact with her she left the Medical Center. The next media article indicated that the medical center was going to criminally charge the nurses, including the head nurse, for the overdose. At this point, I took my documented data over to the medical center and placed the documents directly in the hands of the head nurse. As a result, there was no more talk about any criminal charges. The data that I provide to her indicated that the problem was in the process itself. Two drugs were used to treat the reporter's medical problem. One drug was used to suppress the body's auto immune process so that the second drug could act on the medical problem. When it was observed that the reporter's immune system was not suppressed they prescribed additional dosages of the other drug. This resulted in an overdose of the drug. The reporter, upon autopsy, did not exhibit any medical problems. When this writer returned home, after giving my data to the head nurse, I hardly got my coat off when I received a telephone call from someone allegedly in security, at the medical center, informing me that if I ever set foot in the medical center again that I will be arrested for trespassing.

The next example of Health Care terrorism involves the Mother and Father of the two year old girl and the 500 mg of amoxicillin prescribed for her as outlined in my INTRODUCTION. Despite the fact that both parents were directly involved in the pharmaceutical industry neither one of them questioned the unbelievable dosage of 500 mg of amoxicillin, for a two year old. As a matter of fact, I questioned why the Father did not go to the pharmacist that evening, to pick up the prescription, after he left the pediatricians office. Also, I thought it strange that he wanted me to give the medication to his daughter the next day. The only possible reason for his actions was that he was afraid to question the

500mg of amoxicillin for his daughter for fear of alienating the AMA. and/or the pharmaceutical industry, which he was a part of.

I believe the next example of Health Care Terrorism really points out the power the AMA. and the drug industry have over educational institutions. I went to the then President, and the Dean of the Pharmaceutical College at my alma mater, Northeastern University, and offered to turn over my rights to two proposed medical patents, Medication update software total and Perfect prescription package. These patents are detailed in the chapter on Suggestion and Proposals for a Healthier Life. Despite being familiar with me, since I was a well know athlete at the university and my cooperative work assignment was at the University, their response was nothing but deadly silence. It was obvious to them that, after reviewing my patents, that the implementation of these patents would result in a big loss of money for the medical industry.

The next example involved this writer, personally. I was taking the most dangerous drug on the market, a blood thinner. My doctor kept insisting that I take a stronger dosage so that I would attain the correct INR. ratio. When I attempted to follow up with her request by taking a stronger dose I had adverse auto immune reactions. These reactions are covered in the chapter on Cause and Prevention of Adverse Reactions to Drugs. I attempted to explain my problem to her but she would not listen to me. When I went to the pharmacist to renew my prescription, at a lower dosage, I was informed that I could not obtain it since I no longer had a doctor to approve it, as a result of my doctor cutting me off without notice. Fortunately, I just stopped taking the blood thinner without any problems.

One of the worse cases of health care terrorism among the medical establishment came about from a leading Boston doctor who was the director of an institute for the improvement of health care. I labeled his acts of health care terrorism, as terrorism by deadly silence, since he chose to remain deadly silent while terror prevailed among people from the death and disabilities from medical problems. His game plan was to remain deadly silent by being unavailable to respond to this writer, since he was always unavailable, since he was always out of town. I attempted to thwart his game plan by contacting his aide to set up a time, a place, and a location that I could meet with him. Maybe it was just coincidental or maybe his aide just quit since she did not agree with her doctor's game plan, regardless, she suddenly was no longer the doctor's aide. It was obvious, similar to his colleagues, he could not evaluate my findings on the cause and prevention of medical problems since there is no money in finding the cause and prevention of medical problems.

Possibly, the most significant act on the part of the Health Care Terrorism revolved around the Doctor, Director, Autoimmune Disease Research Center, at a leading University. In an article that he presented for the American Autoimmune Related Diseases Association, Inc. he raised two questions that he sought answers for. First question was: How does autoimmunity arise? What causes the body to produce an immune response to itself? Second question was: What are the factors in the autoimmune response that sometimes causes a disease"? Based on my own personal experience I E mailed the answers to these two questions to him. He never responded to my E mail choosing to allow the Public to be terrorized by the process.

Ironically, the greatest act, of on going acts, of health care terrorism, is the failure on the part of the medical scientific establishment and associated affiliates to provide documented data, to the public, on the body's adverse autoimmune process. I provide details of this process in my chapter, Effects of Body Processes. I cite the failure to provide this information to the Public as a weapon of ongoing terrorism because this process is responsible for the majority of chronic medical problems. With the data in this book I challenge all my many contacts to prove me wrong. In particular I issue my challenge to Congressman Waxman of California, since he is an elected official, who issued a news letter that I received from the Sjogren Syndrome Society referencing autoimmune diseases and Sjogren Syndrome. I detailed the cause and prevention of Sjogren Syndrome in my chapter on Cause and Prevention of Medical problems.

Possibly, the best examples of the fear that the average person has, for health care terrorism, was reflected in the responses of my contacts to my findings on Japan. I played bridge with seniors at the local senior center. As I moved from table to table all I heard was about their medical problems and the drugs that they were taking for these problems. When I returned from a trip to Japan I stood up in front of the about five tables and made an offer. I offered to provide them with data on why Japan is the healthiest nation in the world with no obesity. I suggested that they call me, that I am in the book, and that they don't have to identify themselves. I did not receive a single call. However, what might be even worse was when I would tell future contacts about this response they would all express shock at this response, but would never want to know why Japan is the healthiest nation in the world, with no obesity.

Finally, when ever I provided documented data to any of my contacts, on their particular medical problem, I always had to warn them not to confront anyone in the medical field with this data. Unfortunately, the medical professional will view this act as challenging their authority and will cut them off as their patient. Naturally, they will also notify their colleagues, leaving you without a doctor..

CAUSE AND PREVENTION OF MEDICAL RESEARCH FAILURES

A recent article in the media I believe set the tone for problems with medical research. The article indicated that of the 22 greatest discoveries of the 20th century, 16 were during the first half of the century, and, of the other six, most of the basic research was done prior to 1950. Anti biotics was as a result of basic research. Is it possible that the lack of an immediate return on one's investment is the main cause of the lack of new discoveries, particularly in medicine?

At the present time, there is very little medical research that addresses the cause and prevention of medical problems. At the present time, the approach to solving medical problems, by the medical scientific establishment, is all after the fact with cure and treatment. A medical writer, writing in a Boston newspaper, correctly addressed the problem with our failure to look at solving medical problems from the cause and prevention perspective. She wrote that 90 percent of US healthcare dollars are spent on treating and curing disease, and only one percent on preventing disease. She went on to say that promoting health and averting diseases saves more lives, more cheaply, than does high-tech medicine. In the article she went on to quote a Dr. Julie Gerberding "robust" funding of disease prevention programs could each year save diabetics from 43,000 amputations, 165,000 kidney failures, and more than 10,000 cases of eye disease, reduce by half 40,000 HIV infections and forestall two-thirds of alcohol exposed pregnancies". Also, the medical research associated with the discovery of medications, to address medical problems, leaves much to be desired. Organizations, such as the American cancer society, are straightforward when they solicit for funds indicating that the funds are to help to discover the cure for cancers. For examples of the status of medical research one only has to look at the statements made by the NY. Times, and those of a woman doctor. The NY. Times, in an article on medical problems, indicated that there were plenty of problems (medical) out there but why solve them if there is no money in it. That's right; no company in their right mind would want to spend millions of dollars to find out that if you ate a certain agent that you would not contract connective tissue medical problems. As far as the grants issued by the federal government for research into the cause and prevention of a particular medical problem, this was covered in the same NY. Times article. In a quote by a research Doctor, who said, "if you pay me $50,000, per year, to solve a particular medical problem I will never solve that problem". A women Doctor, with the National Institute of Health, and the wife of a US Congressman, in a leading Women's magazine said. "I am really disturbed with my colleagues, recently, a close friend of mine died of breast cancer and the approach and treatment on my best friend was identical to that of my Mother who died of the same breast cancer 20 years ago". Let's face it, if a Woman no less, with her credentials no less, is unable to alter the failure of medical research what chances does the average person have. This writer made contact with a leading research Doctor, with the National Cancer Society and I asked him how it was possible that a group of (World Wide) so called experts on breast cancer could meet in Boston, recently, and adjourn, without issuing a single statement regarding breast cancer. He responded, "I really don't know I was not invited." That's right just because he was not invited he could care less what, if anything, the breast cancer experts discovered. A young research biochemist, with a leading University in Cambridge Ma., when informed by this writer that I had documented data that non metabolized protein may cause serious medical problems responded, "Wow we all need protein". As far as ongoing medical research, where the researcher obviously was not interested in the cause and prevention of Alzheimer's disease one only has to review this writer's one way correspondence with a leading Boston University. I provided the University with my documented data on the cause and prevention of Alzheimer's disease with no response from them. Two years later I got in touch with this group and asked them if they had any data on their findings, regarding this study. There was a very long pause and the person came back and indicated that they had no data at this time. I then asked when they thought they might have some data. Once again there was a long wait and then the person said not for another three years. There was the epidemiologist who spent two years researching his illness, and two hospital visits before finding out that his illness was caused by a common food colorant. There was the leading Boston heart research specialist that obtained a ten million dollar research grant in January and died of a heart attack, at home, in June, of the same year. Other examples of the failure of proper medical research involved breast cancer. This writer contacted several cancer societies and/or breast cancer foundations and made them an offer. I offered to donate a large sum of money to them if they would provide me with the name of any person and/or persons that they knew that were working on the cause and prevention of breast cancer. No one could provide me with a name. On the internet I was able to obtain a list of the organizations that had NIH research grants involving breast cancer. Out of the 717 organizations referenced only one was working on the cause and prevention of breast cancer. Ironically, that group was looking into genetics as the cause of breast cancer, with genetics as an ongoing research subject among most research groups. In another example of the failure of medical research it involved my responding to an advertisement for volunteers to join a study group on aging. When I received the form to fill out to see if I would qualify for the study I knew that I would not qualify because of the first question. The first question asked if I was allergic to any medications. I responded by informing them that I was allergic to the preservatives in drugs. Later in the form I indicated that I did not require any medications. Naturally, I did not hear back from them since it was obvious that their program called for the taking of drugs to stop aging.

During this writer's fact findings I discovered a catch 22 situation within the non profit medical research groups. If the for profit medical research groups reluctantly accepted this writer's findings, on the possible cause and prevention of a medical problem, they were still in business. However, if the nonprofit medical research groups accepted my findings on the cause and prevention of their medical problem, specialty, they were immediately out of business.

Americans have as much say over the direction and technology of medical research as they do over who should be the king of Tonga. Per usual, the American approach is that anything can be solved by the influx of money. It is obvious that this approach has not worked since, despite spending billions on researching breast cancer, no one is close to finding the cure and/or the cause of breast cancer. Within our democratic process the widest gap between public participation and our government is in medical research. The scientific establishment controls the depth and types of medical research. Unknown to most Americans nearly half the funding for our medical research comes from the Federal Government, through the National Institute of Health (NIH). The NIH., sponsoring of medical research is unique as government spending goes, because the NIH. allocates funds not according to some central plan, but rather responds to the advice of the applicants peers from the scientific grass roots that review individual proposals. Once the research grant is made, the recipient only has to publish some data, any data, regardless if it is truly material to solving the medical problem in question. By keeping the information flowing into the NIH, the money will continue to flow from the NIH.. Congress has seen fit to place money for medical research at the bottom of the budget requests. Only one in five research projects, considered important, are funded. Unfortunately, Congress is locked in deficit reduction madness and has failed to provide the NIH with sufficient funding to meet the necessary medical research projects.

During my fact finding I found that children and Women were not being fairly treated when it came to medical research. I believe that an article in the Baltimore Sun summed it up when it reported that health care groups say drugs are not tested for use on children. In regard to women, the medical researchers are only able to make statements without any follow up. For example, the Reuters article said researchers find increase peril for young women. A study was made of 90,000 women ages 26 to 46 over eight years and during this period 714 developed invasive breast cancer. In the article it stressed that young women who ate red meat and full-fat dairy products such as cheese raised their risks of contracting breast cancer. I wish it was that simple. A review of the data on medical problems with menopause says it all. Also, the media article on the lack of testing of drugs' on women often unknown, supports my findings that women are not treated fairly. This writer believes that medical research on the cause and prevention of breast cancer should follow up on the findings of Jehovah. Jehovah said to Moses I have heard the murmurs of the children of Israel tell them to eat bread in the morning and flesh at night. When Jehovah referred to bread he was talking about starch and when he referred to flesh he was talking about red meat. In modern terms if one eats too much starch at the same time as they eat too much red meat the pancreas can't metabolize the protein in the red meat and the protein in the red meat may turn toxic and attack the body cells. The chemical involved is called cytolysin. Similar to children, women have problems with drugs as a result of the lack of proper testing. The media article indicated that 75% of those individuals affected by autoimmune diseases were women (see definition of auto immune process in chapter on body processes). The article in" Today's Woman" listed a few autoimmune diseases such as Lupus, Thyroid, Multiple sclerosis, and Rheumatoid arthritis that they referred to as all women's mystery diseases. They trigger vague, hard to pin down symptoms, such as fatigue, joint pain, rashes, or tingling limbs, all of which may be attributed to emotional upset. This writer feels that these medical problems are more evident, at times, within women because of the uniqueness of the female body with the vagina, and the bartholin glands, with vaginal lubricants and bacterial balance problems. Also, when a woman is pregnant every thing she ingests passes by the placenta. Also, in my personal opinion, a woman's body reacts unlike a man's to particular factors of the body's autoimmune process. These factors are the accumulation, compounding, and or the synergetic, of all ingested agents and/or substances. As far as children are concerned, in all fairness to the medical researchers, since a child's body is in a constant changing mode, it is virtually impossible to conduct any long term medical research on a child's body.

As indicated within my documented data, one of the body's most important body processes is the body's auto immune process (AIP). Unfortunately, the body's adverse reaction to what it considers is a foreign agent and/or substance to the body may result in a serious medical problem, sometimes even a chronic medical problem. For an example: of how the medical scientific establishment (MSE) fails to properly address the above one only has to review the media article, put out by AP., on 12-26-06. The title of the article was "Study Attempts to Trump Food Allergies". The source of the article had a doctor's name on it. In the article it stressed that the peanut could be a food allergy for some people, and it cited the history of a young girl. While in the article it noted that the reaction to the peanut was called an allergy, they cited examples of the more serious adverse auto immune reaction, on the part of the young girl. The article went on to say that one of the participants, in the study, took epinephrine with her to any party to allow the chaperone "to use an a shot of epinephrine, to resist any life threatening reaction." In the article they were going around and around in regard to how many peanuts some of their study participants could take without an allergic reaction (their words not mine). This writer is on record, in my documented data, that at times it was not the agent and/or substance itself that gave me an adverse auto immune reaction, but the quantity. In addition to the above they compounded the problem with their lack of knowledge of the actual autoimmune reaction chemistry. They indicated that a person had an allergic reaction to an allergen when they described an auto immune reaction to an antigen.

I am sorry, I don't feel that there is any excuse why, in 2007, members of the medical profession don't know the difference between the less severe allergic reactions versus the more severe adverse auto immune reactions. In my younger days I would have sent the doctor, referenced, a copy of the medical definition of an allergic reaction versus an autoimmune reaction. However, today if I sent this document to the doctor they would probably sue me.

While the NIH. is the prime mover within the medical research process, relative to finding the cause and prevention of medical problems, it is the FDA that is the prime mover in determining what little medical research exists among the drug companies regarding cure and treatment of medical problems. Unfortunately, the Wall ST. Journal reported that the drug companies may be hiding the data on their drug trials. The reporting process involves voluntary reporting of any negative findings on any drugs by the drug companies. Once again both children and women are not treated fairly. About three-quarters of the drugs prescribed to American children have not had adequate pediatric trials. An accidental ingestion of one pill or a teaspoon of a certain drugs may be toxic enough to cause the death of a 22-pound child. Although women make up just over half of all visits to the doctor's office they receive 73 % of all prescriptions written for psychotropic medications, and an incredible 90%, when the doctor is not a psychiatrist. Women receive up to 83% of prescriptions for antidepressants, well in excess of the 66% that would be expected based on the 2-1 female to male ratio for depression. Overall women have twice as many fatal drug reactions as men. More than twice as many women as men enter the emergency room for adverse reactions to antidepressants. It was found that women respond more slowly than men do to antidepressants: four weeks for women, versus two for men. As far as after the fact medical research is concerned its success has been limited. I believe that a recent media article pointed out why we need more research in this area. The article indicated that for many patients' targeted therapies have been disappointments. Researchers found that tumors seem to have more pathways than field mice in a meadow. In breast cancer alone, there are at least two dozen. One should consider the possibility of how, just a limited knowledge, on how cells become cancerous, might make targeted therapies successful.

Meanwhile, the partial medical research, all after the fact, by the drug companies has developed a novel approach to medical research. Since the 1960's drug companies appear to have developed a medication first and then along comes the disease. Per a doctor at the University of Toronto, he feels that "the drug industry has played a much greater role in shaping our understanding of psychiatric illnesses then previously acknowledged", however, this is not medical research. As a result, the drug companies find themselves missing the dangers of some drugs because of the failure of proper research..

This writer believes that if the MSE does resolve to enter into pure medical research their success in determining the cause and prevention of medical problems will be determined by their knowledge of two key body processes. These processes are the body's autoimmune and autonomic as defined in the chapter on body processes. In particular, it is the body's adverse reaction to these processes. If one eliminates medical problems from genetics, virus, and/or bacterial infections it leaves medical problems caused by the body's adverse autoimmune and/or autonomic reactions as the prime cause of chronic medical problems. Unfortunately, the MSE identifies the body's auto immune processes as an allergic reaction. During my many years of collecting data on the above body process I continued to make excuses for the MSE for their use of the term allergy when it was obvious it was an autoimmune reaction. I believed that the MSE used the allergy term because it was easier for their patient to understand this process since the auto immune process was more complicated. However, as I continued to collect data on this process I realized that in many cases the MSE did not properly understand the body's autoimmune process so they relied on the term allergy. The next key unaddressed auto immune problems involved this writer and Sjogren Syndrome (SS).(see chapter on cause and prevention of medical problems). The MSE admits that they don't know what causes it and therefore they don't know how to treat it. They believe that it is associated with the body's autoimmune process. The SS disorder was discovered by a Swedish doctor. Since this writer found the cause and prevention of my Sjogren Syndrome problem I attempted to contact the SS Society in Sweden. I went through the Swedish Consultant in Boston. Through the consultant I received two documents sent to them by the SS society in Sweden. The first document provided data on the SS Society in Sweden. It was in Swedish which meant very little to me. I physically went to Sweden hoping to visit with the SS. Syndrome society. I found that the location address was nothing but a mailing address. Along with this document I received another document that caught this writer by surprise. I received a document, published by US. Congressman Waxman, of California, indicating that he was proposing a House bill HP2577 to study the autoimmune process. I attempted to contact Representative Waxman in order to provide him with documented data that would prove that the cause of SS is the body's adverse autoimmune process. He never responded to my faxes. Also, I never heard another word about the proposed H.P. 2573 bill involving the autoimmune diseases. I believe that at this point the reader might consider that it was just a coincidence that this writer could not find anyone in the MSE that would properly address the body's autoimmune process.

This writer believes that in order for the reader to fully appreciate the various medical problems, that this writer feels needs a lot of medical research, it is necessary for the reader to familiarize themselves with the body's inflammation process. As I have indicated through out my writings I feel that the key too many medical problems is the requirement to properly address the body's auto immune process which in itself is the inflammation process. I believe that one look at the key points in the Time magazine article on inflammation says it all. "Inflammation is the body's first defense against infection, but when it goes awry, it can lead to heart attacks, colon cancer, Alzheimer's and a host of other diseases" "Scientists are starting to see links to an age old immunological defense mechanism called inflammation, with the same biological process that causes swelling in an injured toe and other illnesses. Everywhere they turn Doctors are finding evidence that inflammation plays a larger role in chronic diseases then they thought. However, that doesn't necessarily mean they know what to do about it. "Were in a quandary right now" says a doctor, an immunologist, at the University of Texas Medical School at Houston. "We're advancing the idea to heighten awareness",. "but we really can't recommend specific treatments yet" "When immune cells get called in they bring growth factors and a whole slew of proteins that call in other inflammatory cells" "Those things come in and go heal, heal," "But instead of healing you're feeding, feeding, feeding" "Sometimes the reason for the initial inflammatory cycle is obvious as with chronic heartburn which continually bathes the lining of the esophagus with stomach acid predisposing a person to esophageal cancer". "Other times it's less clear". Scientists are exploring the role of an enzyme called cyclo-oxygenase @ (cox-2) in the development of colon cancer. Cox-2 is yet another protein produced by the body during inflammation. Inflammation may be more of a problem in the earlier stages of autoimmune diseases like multiple sclerosis. So much tissue is eventually destroyed that nerve damage becomes permanent. "Your initial goal is to keep the immune response in check, but then you have to ask how you encourage regrowth of damaged tissue" says a Doctor, vice president for research programs, at the National Multiple Sclerosis Society. It could take decades to figure that one out. Back in the 1860s renowned pathologist Rudolf Virchow speculated that cancerous tumors arise at the site of chronic inflammation. A century later oncologists paid more attention to the role that various genetic mutations play in promoting abnormal growths that eventually become malignant. Now researchers are exploring the possibility that mutually reinforced processes, that left unchecked, can transform normal cells into potentially deadly tumors. It is believed that in Alzheimer's, the glial cells in the brain that are suppose to support neurons in an attempt to return things to normal, release too many cytokines, that trigger greater cell destruction. But for some reason, in neurodegenerative diseases like Alzheimer's, the process seems to be out of control. You get chronic glial activation, which results in an inflammatory state. Satins are being tested for their anti-inflammatory effects on Alzheimer's disease and sickle cell anemia. Not to long ago most doctors thought of heart attacks as primarily a plumbing problem. Over the years, fatty deposits would slowly build up on the insides of major coronary arteries until they grew so big that they cut off the supply of blood to a vital part of the heart. Supposedly, the bad cholesterol provided the raw material for these deposits. There's just one problem with that explanation, sometimes its dead wrong. Half of all heart attacks occur in people with normal cholesterol levels. Doctor's found that much to their surprise, that the most dangerous plaques weren't necessarily all that large. In the 1990s Doctors became convinced that some sort of inflammatory reaction was responsible for the bursting plaque. At the same time Doctor's found that for whatever reason the cytokine signals began ramping up the inflammatory process instead of notching it down, so the plaque became unstable. One of the most intriguing questions in immunology today is why everyone doesn't suffer from asthma. After all, the air we breathe is full of germs, viruses and other irritants. Americans with asthma are hyper sensitive to common substances like cat dander or pollen. It stands to reason that their allergic reactions trigger the chronic inflammation in their bodies. Yet the people who develop asthma as adults, one of the most rapidly growing segment of the population, often don't have allergies.

While this writer in this chapter attempts to concentrate on the cause and prevention of medical problems, medical research must continue with the cure and treatment process with the research of drugs. Unfortunately, the Wall Street Journal reported that studies showing negative results, involving drugs, often go unpublished. The Journal reported that there is black hole in drug medical research where as many as half of all drug studies, especially ones with negative results, remain unpublished. An editor in chief of the New England Journal of Medicine, says that" many drug trials are designed to show that one medicine isn't any worse than another". "While this approach reduces the number of patients and money needed to test a medicine, it often undercuts the ability of investigators to draw valid conclusions about side effects or other clinical questions". Also, a major source of the problem starts with the researchers themselves. There tends to be a bias in all of science, not just medicine, to publish positive results rather than negative results. Finally, in many cases the pharmaceutical industry controls their own drug research. In many cases the FDA is forced, by the drug companies, to approve a drug without the necessary long term research.

The major medical problems requiring a break through in finding the cause and prevention of these medical problems are the cancers particularly Breast cancer, Diabetes,(D), particularly type two found in children, Alzheimer's, Asthma, diseases of the colon, diseases of the eyes, and diseases associated with the pancreas. Breast cancer medical research should concentrate on the auto immune process producing cytoysin that attacks and destroys the breast cells. The breast cancer researchers should look at the cause and prevention of breast cancer in Massachusetts since Massachusetts led the nation in female breast cancer and

Hodgkin's disease rates. In a media article it mentioned the possible reason for the high Hodgkin's disease rate. It stated that the high Hodgkin's disease rate may be related to the Bay State's affluence. A study found that higher socioeconomic groups have, for reasons unknown, higher Hodgkin's disease rates. The article went on to say Jewish women, for reasons unknown, have higher than average breast cancer rates.

Diabetes (D) In an article in Time magazine it cited that never have Doctors known so much about how to prevent or control this disease, yet the epidemic continues. In the article it stated that any scientist who can figure out why Type 2 diabetics are insulin resistant will probably be a candidate for a Nobel Prize. Diabetes (D) is characterized as a failure of carbohydrates to metabolize. Usually it is a genetic problem and/or from the inadequate production and/or utilization of insulin that results in excessive amounts of glucose in the blood.. Type1 (D) is a severe form of (D) in which insulin production by the beta cells of the pancreas are impaired. Type 2 (D) is characterized by a diminished tissue sensitivity to insulin and sometimes impaired beta cell function. In the same article it touched upon the possibility that the inflammation caused by an adverse autoimmune reaction may increase a person's risk of developing Type 2 diabetes. This writer feels that medical research on the cause and prevention of diabetes naturally has to center around two key body organs. The liver, which releases a controlled amount of glucose, and the pancreas, that releases a controlled amount of insulin. This writer believes that the amounts of these two chemicals that are released are directly affected by the body's adverse auto immune reaction that reduces and/or blocks entirely these two chemicals. Once again the MSE must properly address the body's autoimmune process if they are to properly address the reason why so many people are getting diabetes. At the same time the researchers must study the possible requirement to replace metabolic enzymes lost as a result of genetic problems and/or enzymes blocked by the adverse auto immune process. There also is a need to replace any hormones lacking from the beta cells of the pancreas.

Alzheimers The Chicago-based Alzheimer's Association has funded a research project that has zeroed in on the beta amyloid protein as a key to the Alzheimer's disease. This writer believes that researchers should look at the process where the body has an autoimmune reaction that directly affects the digestive enzymes starting in the mouth. This causes the person to fail to properly metabolize starch. This unmetabolized starch turns into an insoluble super plaque or beta amyloid. that clog's the arteries to the brain

Asthma The article in the Wall Street Journal reported that the National Academy of Science found that people exposed to indoor mold develop asthma.

Also the indoor mold in conjunction with other ingested agents and/or substances causes the inflammation of the respiratory tract. All research on asthma should concentrate on the cause and prevention of asthma by the elimination of indoor mold.

Sense of balance The article in the media was titled Volunteers aid researchers studying balance. Per usual within the article it stressed that research was being conducted to develop balance enhancing devices. This is all after the fact. In fact the Massachusetts Ear and Eye Infirmary have a $2.5 million federal grant to develop a balance enhancing vest or belt. This writer suggests that the balancing problems described in this article is as a result of an adverse auto immune reaction that causes the inner ear canal to become swollen causing the disruption of the inner ear fluid that controls balance, hence vertigo. This process should be researched to find the cause and prevention of this adverse auto immune reaction. As indicated in the media article, some people have balance problems from an auto immune reaction to some drugs. The article stressed that one person had her worse bouts of vertigo at the grocery store. In this writer's opinion this is caused by the cross over process within the body's auto immune process involving mold/fungus in the air.

Macular degeneration (MD) The status of MD research is reflected in the facts and stats indicated below.. A Richard Rosen was quoted "We can't cure MD but we may be able to halt the progression of blindness". "There are two types of MD the dry type which rarely leads to blindness and the "wet" type which is far more dangerous". In the wet form an abnormal number of blood vessels begin rapidly growing at the back of the eye, just behind the retina. These vessels usually begin to leak. Research has centered on preventing this leakage. A Doctor Snodderly is investigating two yellow pigments; known as carotenoids that are concentrated in the macula. These pigments, lutein and zeaxanthin are taken into the blood stream through the diet. Another study is focusing on the build up of a cellular waste product in the eye, lipofuscin and how to get rid of this substance. This study is in patients where the researchers are able to relate to the amount of lipofuscin to the progression of aging. Once again I would like to suggest to the researchers that they study the cause and prevention of the build up of lipofuscin in the first place. Researchers believe that lipofuscin is a product of oxidative damage to cells. Normal cellular processes can generate different forms of reactive oxygen that damage cellular molecules. In my contact with the Schepens Eye Research Institute I believe that their response says it all. In the letter in response to my letter to them they said. I spoke with a Doctor, and she says you are right when you point out that lipofuscin build-up is not the initial cause of retinal damage. The first level of damage is indeed due to oxidation. The letter went on to address some of my other concerns. Researchers are studying the goal of preventing the initial oxidative damage through harnessing protective substances in the diet. Once again they must study the lack of oxygen as a result of the body's adverse autoimmune reaction. In addition to the above, research should go forward on the protein called Labaudinere that is known to cause nerodegegeneration in parkinson's disease. Researchers are hoping to discover a drug that will eliminate this protein. Also, there is a disease know as familial amyloid cardiomyopathy that causes heart failure. The process causes a protein to misfold and researchers are looking for treatment to prevent the misfolding of the protein.

Researchers are close to discovering a super antibiotic that stimulates the white blood cells that in turn attacks bacteria. Supposedly this protein stimulates the immune cells to release the antimicrobial compound to kill bacteria.

Scientists are close to discovering on how cells unite to allow for the spread of cancers. The process involved is called metastasis, however it is an area of medicine that scientists have not been very successful in discovering details on the process involved.

The spore producing bacterium Clostridium Difficile also known as C-diff., is becoming more of a menace in hospitals and nursing homes. The bacteria are spread by spores in the feces and these bacteria have been difficult to kill.

The French think that they have discovered the cause of Sudden Respiratory Syndrome (SARS). At the present time the discovery only involves mice.

The British medical journal, reported, that they think they have found the cause of Crohn"s disease. They are investigating a bacterium called Mycobacterium that may be the cause of Crohn"s disease.

Germany is well on it's way to developing an enzyme replacement program, however, the US should not wait for their results.

The Associated Press reported on 12-14-05 that the NIH had established a $100 million project to speed up the discovery of what causes genes to run amok and cause cancers. Finally, this writer believes that the goal of this research project is the ultimate in medical research. This writer hopes that the researchers will investigate the body's adverse auto immune reaction on the body's cells along with investigating the adverse, reverse, toxic protein reaction on the body's cells. In both cases this reaction may cause the cells to go amok and/or become destroyed.

Separate from the above, but in conjunction with the above, is the report of research on a vaccine for cancer. Hans-Werner, founder of German software giant SAP AG, will offer Therion Biologics Corp., $50 million to develop a vaccine for cancer within the next two years. Naturally, this drastically changes the treatment approach to preventing cancers.

EFFECTS OF BODY PROCESSES

As you review the effects of key body processes keep in mind that the body, with its various processes, is like a complicated machine. As a result of the many complicated body processes the key body processes are not always properly understood and/or addressed by the medical establishment (ME). For example: the ME uses one word, allergy, to identify the less serious medical problems with an allergy, versus the more serious medical problems with an adverse autoimmune reaction. An allergy occurs when the body develops a specific antibody, to a specific antigen. Meanwhile, an adverse autoimmune reaction takes place when the body reacts, to an antigen, by attacking the body itself. The body's autoimmune process acts normally when it reacts to an antigen, by attacking the body. This is an attempt by the body to defend itself against what the body considers as a foreign agent, thereby causing medical problems. Also, the autoimmune process may adversely affect other body processes. Most important, the ME may incorrectly diagnose the autoimmune reaction as an infection and incorrectly prescribe medications, which not only compounds the problem, but the medication in itself, may cause an adverse autoimmune reaction.

Autoimmune process

Cytokines The body's autoimmune process involves a class of proteins called inflammation cytokines * that adversely affects the liquid glands of the body that includes the pancreas, liver, saliva, and the bladder. I believe the article in Time magazine titled The Fires Within says it all. "Inflammation is the body's first defense against infection, but when it goes awry, it can lead to heart attacks, colon cancer, Alzheimer's and a host of other diseases". Unfortunately, the article is wrong in saying it goes awry since its actions are normal. The cytokine acts similar to an antibody and attempts to defend the body against what the body perceives as a foreign agent and/or substance within in the air, food, drink, and/ or medications. It is possible to have more than one adverse reaction at the same time from more than one trigger. This process is activated by the body ingesting a type of antigen (protein) that under the appropriate conditions is capable of inducing a specific immune response and of reacting with the product of that response. The response is characterized by a specific humeral element (an element, protein) that dissolves in the blood cells or body fluids. It forms a type of antibody within the blood (autoimmune) as opposed to the antibody associated with a regular cellular type (allergy). As a result, the body responds against constituents of its own body tissues (attacks its own body). Also, there is an autoimmune reaction called cross over where the body is unable to tell the difference between a good agent and a bad agent. For example: the body is unable to tell the difference between good yeast, a fungi, and a bad fungus and may adversely react to both. This process involves the body's adverse reaction to the accumulation, compounding, and/or synergetic, of certain ingested agents and/or substances within the air, food, drink, and/or medications. In this process the liquid glands of the body are inflamed and/or swollen thereby blocking and/or reducing the flow of enzymes necessary for the body's metabolic/digestive process. These key enzymes that are secreted from the pancreas, are the protease, ** that breaks down protein, amylase that breaks down carbohydrates, lipase that breaks down fats, and cellulose, that breaks down fiber. Compounding the above digestive process is the part that genetics play involving digestive enzyme secretions. The process is regulated by two factors neural and hormonal. Neural control is usually based on the body sensing a physical mass of food. This stimulation generally results from a stretching of the digestive tract. Meanwhile, smelling, tasting, and even thinking about food stimulates the salivary and some gastric enzyme secretions. Hormonal control is more specific. The presence of specific kinds of molecules in the ingested foods, themselves, stimulates receptor cells to produce a specific hormone. The hormone circulates in the blood until it reaches the secreting organ, which it controls. The above process, less digestive/metabolic enzymes, means medical problems. The initial body's auto immune reaction is usually slow to react and not too intense. However, each subsequent body contact with a foreign agent and/or substance results in a quicker reaction and a more intense reaction. Possibly, a prime example as to how the body reacts, under the above circumstances, took place with this writer and titanium dioxide. I was having a salad with fresh vegetables and mayonnaise for a dressing. I immediately had to run to the bathroom more than once to urinate. Realizing that it was an autoimmune reaction I could not understand what was triggering my body's autoimmune process. Finally, I turned the pickle jar around and read the section on ingredients and found my answer, it was titanium dioxide put in the pickle jar as a preservative. I called up the product manager, for a well known pickle manufacture, and asked him why he would put the strongest preservative on the market, titanium dioxide, in pickles that were in vinegar, that you were told to refrigerate after opening. I believe his response said it all" to maintain the color".

This writer is able to create an autoimmune reaction, not only by what I ingest, but also by the quantity of what I ingest.

Naturally, during the above processes medications may not be metabolized. These medications in turn may cause their own adverse body reactions as a result of an overdose.

CYTOKININ* any of a class of phytohormones (A) whose principle functions are the induction of cell division and the regulation of differentiation of tissues. **CYTOKINE** a generic term for non-antibody proteins released by one cell population on contact with a specific antigen, which acts as intercellular mediators, as in the generation of an immune response. (examples include lymphokines (B) and monokines) (C) **CYTOLYSIS** the dissolution or destruction of cells. **CYTOKINESIS** the changes that take place in the cytoplasm during the cell division, a process synchronized in eukaryotic cells with nuclear division (mitosis)./A/is a combining form of hormones/B/is any lymphocyte product, as interferon (D) that is not an antibody but may participate in the immune response through it's effect on the function of other cells, as destroying antigen coated cells, or stimulating macrophages (E)./C/is any substance secreted by a monocyte (F) or macrophage and affecting the function of other cells./D/is any of various proteins produced by virus infected cells that inhibit reproduction of the invading virus and induce resistance to further infection./E/is a large white blood cell occurring principally in connective tissue and in the blood stream that ingests foreign particles and infectious micro organism by phagocytosis (G)./F/is a large circulating white blood cell formed in bone marrow and in the spleen that ingests large foreign particles and cell debris./G/is ingestion of a smaller cell or foreign particles by in folding the of cell's membrane and protrusion of its cytoplasm around the fold until material has been engulfed by closure of the membrane and formation of a vacuole: characteristic of some type of white blood cells. **CYTOL-YSIN** a substance, or a type of an antibody, that causes the destructions of cells. **LYSOME** (L) a minute body in many types of cells containing various hydrolytic enzymes that are involved in localized intracellular digestion. Injury to the (L) causes the release into the cell of the enzymes which may damage the cells causing certain diseases such as breast cancer.

PROTEASE any of a group of enzymes, that catalyze the hydrolytic degradation of proteins and/or polypeptides to smaller amino acid polymers.

As the reader reviews the body's autoimmune process it should become obvious that this important body function may seriously affect the body's autonomic process.

Special note*The pepsin that is involved in this process may only function in a highly acidic medium which must be maintained for several hours in order to complete the metabolism of the protein.

The American Autoimmune Related Disease Association claims that as a result of the above autoimmune responses several so-called autoimmune diseases are contracted. They claim that there are two major factors that cause these diseases, genetics and environmental. They go on to say that autoimmune diseases are not typical genetic diseases. Multiple genes are involved in the autoimmune disease process, not a specific gene, such as in sickle cell anemia. This writer found that the one common denominator is that the process involves the inflammation of the body's liquid glands, and/or body tissue. This inflammation reaction is caused by an adverse autoimmune reaction to what the body considered to be a foreign agent and/or substance. Time magazine I believe summed it up in an article titled THE FIRES WITHIN. In the article it stated inflammation is the body's first defense against infection, but when it goes awry, it can lead to heart attacks, colon cancer, Alzheimer's and a host of other diseases.

Synergism

This process is one of those associated processes that, in conjunction with the body's autoimmune process, may cause medical problems. Synergism is the inter action of elements that when combined produce a total effect that is greater than the sum of the effects of the individual elements. Originally, I did not consider synergism a key body process. I merely saw this process as a by product of the body's adverse autoimmune process. While it is within the body's overall auto immune process a further look indicates to this writer that it should stand alone as a key body process. In particular, I discovered a process called rhinitis, which ties in with the synergism process. At first I treated the rhinitis process as a medical problem and fully intended to place the write up within my chapter on medical problems. However, at this point I had a personal medical problem, that to this writer was obviously rhinitis, and I realized that rhinitis was not just a simple medical problem, per se, but a factor associated with the body's adverse allergic and/or autoimmune process. Up to this point, medical people referred to the above process as a cross over within the body's autoimmune process. That is to say that the body's auto immune process is unable to distinguish between a good yeast agent and a bad fungi agent and reacts adversely to both. In this case the two agents are from the same plant family, but this is not always necessary in order to experience the cross over process. I also found that this process could occur with other than agents from the same plant family. For example: there is Rhinitis Medicamentous which is a reaction to two or more medications. The most significant example was my first encounter with the above process. While in a production plant I had an adverse reaction to polyurethane foam, which had as one of its chemicals isocyanine, a component of poison gas. Subsequent to that exposure, to those chemicals, I developed adverse reactions to agents and substances that never affected me before. In my own personal experience, leading up to my discovery of the Rhinitis process, I had adverse reactions to the yeast in cookies. Later when I opened the sealed metal box with aged newsprint articles, and other aged printed papers my nose immediately began to run so fast that I didn't have time to reach up and catch the flow. For another example of the above process I would like to cite what I call the super market syndrome. I went into a super market; right after it opened in the morning, and went right to the dairy section. Once in the dairy section I had an adverse reaction to the mold/fungus in the dairy section. Within the same time frame I visited with the head baker on the very opposite end of the store and received an adverse reaction from the yeast at the bakery. This writer found that only after my body purged the initial reactive agent, yeast, did I stop the Synergism process. While I never experienced problems with this process, involving medications, to me it is obvious that among some people the use of medications could compound this problem.`

Autonomic process

This process, as noted, is basically uncontrollable. As a result, it is affected adversely by the functioning of the body's autoimmune process. The autonomic process involves the body's ability to function independently without outside influence, wherein, the nervous system regulates vital functions of the body, which are not consciously controlled (involuntary)! It includes the activity of the heart, the smooth muscles, (such as digestive muscles) and the glands. It has two divisions, the sympathetic nervous system speeds up the heart rate, narrows blood vessels, and raises blood pressure! The parasympathetic nervous system slows the heart rate, increases internal and gland activities, and relaxes ring like muscles, which close passages (sphincters) (see peripheral nervous system). Autonomic reflexes are any of a large number of normal reflexes that regulate the functions of the body's organs. Autonomic reflexes control activities such as blood pressure, heart rate, intestinal activities, sweating and urination. The parasympathetic process releases the chemical acetycholine, an acetic acid ester of choline, which is released and hydrolyzed during nerve conduction. It allows for messages to travel from one nerve to another, resulting in muscle action, by transmitting nerve impulses across the synapse (a enzyme acetylcholine searase) where nerve impulses are transmitted and received, encompassing the axon terminal of a neuron (small gap). Simply put, it allows for a message to the hand to pick up a pen etc. It also activates the peristalsis, wave like rhythmic contractions of the smooth muscles. It forces food through the digestive track, bile through the bile duct, and urine through the urethra. It also releases fluids from the tear, saliva, and digestive glands. It also begins the release of bile and insulin, widens some blood vessels, and relaxes muscles during urination and defecation!

The above process is a necessary adjunct to the body's autoimmune process! In the event that the body has an adverse autoimmune reaction, during certain autonomic processes, serious medical problems may develop!

Breathing/respiratory

In order to understand the respiration process it is necessary to note the difference between breathing and respiration. Respiration has two meanings. First, that it is the oxidative degradation of nutrients such as glucose through metabolic reactions within the cell resulting in the production of carbon dioxide, water and energy. Secondly, it is the exchange of gases between the cells of an organism and the external environment. Breathing may be defined as the mechanical process of taking in air into the lungs (inspiration) and expelling gasses between the blood stream and the alveoli. Breathing requires the coordinated contractions, and relaxations of several muscles. This is achieved by the respiratory center, which is composed of special groups of cells in the medulla and pons of the brain. From this respiratory center, nerve impulses are rhythmically discharged to the intercostals (rib) muscles, resulting in their periodic contraction every 4 to 5 seconds. The breathing movements are automatic and under normal conditions occur without voluntary control. We can voluntarily hold our breath, but not indefinitely, since then the automatic center eventually takes over and forces us to exhale. Respiration is controlled at any time by multiple factors. For example if a person hyperventilates before holding their breath, and then does strenuous exercise the following reactions take place. Hyperventilation causes CO_2 to be lost from the blood faster than it is produced by the cells of the body. This decreased CO_2 levels inhibits the firing of chemo receptors, and the respiratory rate tends to decrease. If a person then holds their breath and exercises, O_2 is lost, but CO_2 will not increase fast enough to stimulate respiration. The connections between the inspiration and expiration centers are inhibitory in nature. At the beginning of inspiration, when the inspiration neurons are firing the expiration is inhibited. When inspiration ceases, expiration inhibition also stops and expiration is able to take place which then, in turn inhibits inspiration. Respiration is stimulated by other factors such as extreme temperatures, pain, initiation of exercise, and certain drugs.

The blood oxygen heart equation

When I found myself unable to breathe correctly while laying down I found myself having to sit up in order to breathe normally! As a result, I went to the emergency room of the hospital! They found that my hematocrit (% of red blood cell count to total blood count) was 19.6% when it should have been 43%. The normal range for women is 37% to 43% and for men it is 43% to 49%. Eryhrocyte contains hemoglobin; its main function is to transport oxygen, which is carried by the hemoglobin. Hemoglobin carries oxygen to the cells, from the lungs and carbon dioxide away from the cells, to the lungs. Oxygen transport is the way oxygen is absorbed in the lungs, by the hemoglobin in red blood cells, and carried to tissue cells all over the body. This process is possible because hemoglobin is able to combine with large amounts of oxygen when it is at high levels, as in the lungs, and to release this oxygen when the oxygen level is low, as in the body tissues. 98% of oxygen is transported by hemoglobin, and the amount of C_2O present controls the combination of hemoglobin and oxygen! Hemoglobin is a complex protein, iron compound, in the blood with 98% oxygen transported by hemoglobin. Carbon hemoglobin is the key to the ratio of carbon to oxygen in the blood. Myoglobin, a protein, is a reserve supply of oxygen and is released when blood pressure is low. Toxins in the blood interfere with the oxygen carrying capacity of the red blood cells. Any increase of C_2O in the blood stimulates an increase in the pulse rate and thus the cardiac output. Also, the change in the blood composition alters the depth and frequency of breathing.

Hemoglobin process

Red blood cells, erythrocyte, contain hemoglobin a complex compound in the blood that carries oxygen to the cells from the lungs and CO_2 away from the cells to the lungs. It serves to transport 98% of the body's oxygen. In the lungs oxygen enters the capillaries and diffuses into the red blood cells where it binds to hemoglobin. Failure of this process results in unfavorable carboxyl hemoglobin.

Electrolyte process

Electrolyte is any solution (potassium, magnesium, & calcium) capable of conducting any electric current by the movement of its disassociated positive and negative ions to the electrode. The element carries as electric charge! The body must correctly process the correct amounts of energy! Calcium relaxes the heart muscles and contracts the heartbeat! Potassium is needed to contract heart muscles and to relax the heart! Sodium is needed to maintain overall fluid balance. Failure of the process means irregular heartbeats!

Circulatory

The circulatory system works closely with the body's respiratory system. The circulatory system consists of the heart, blood vessels, and lymph vessels through which the blood and lymph circulates. Circulation time is the time it takes for the blood to flow from one point of the body to another. Associated with the respiratory/circulation process is the hemoglobin process. The hemoglobin process is where red blood cells, erythrocytres contain hemoglobin a complex iron compound in the blood that carries oxygen to the cells from the lungs and CO_2 away from the cells to the lungs. It serves to transport 98% of the body's oxygen. In the lungs, oxygen enters the capillaries, and diffuses into the red blood cells where it binds to hemoglobin. Hemoglobin thus acts to pick up oxygen where it is available and releases it where it is needed. Myoglobin, on the other hand, has a higher affinity for oxygen than does hemoglobin. Thus, even at relatively low partial pressures, myoglobin still tends to bind with oxygen. Any toxins in the blood may interfere with the oxygen carrying capacity of the red blood cells. The above provides data on circulatory failure which is the inability of the heart and blood vessels (cardiovascular system) to supply enough blood to meet the needs of the cells. Naturally this failure may be caused by an abnormal function of the heart and/or insufficient blood supply in the body.

Digestive process

Digestion is the breakdown of large, ingested molecules into smaller, simple ones that can be absorbed and used by the body. The breakdown of these large molecules is called degradation. During degradation, some of the chemical bonds that hold the large molecules together are split. The digestive enzymes cleave molecular bonds by a process called hydrolysis. In hydrolysis a water molecule is added across the bond to cleave it. Digestion begins in the mouth. Most foods contain polysaccharides such as starch, which are long chains of sugar molecules. The salivary glands in the mouth consist of three pairs of glands. The parotid glands located in the cheek in front of the ear produce only watery saliva, which dissolves dry foods. The sub maxillary and sublingual glands located at the base of the jaw and under the tongue produce watery and mucous saliva, which coagulates food particles, and also lubricate the throat for the passage of lumps of chewed food. Saliva also contains amylase, which break down starches. The enzyme pepsin in the stomach splits the long protein into shorter fragments or peptides that are further digested in the intestines. The acidity of the stomach inhibits the actions of the salivary amylase leaving most of the starch undigested. It is not until the starch reaches the small intestines that another amylase secreted by the pancreas finishes the cleavage of starch into maltose. The tongue pushes the food into the pharynx. The act of swallowing initiates the movement of food down through a tube connecting the mouth to the stomach called the esophagus. Once inside the esophagus the food is moved by involuntary peristaltic waves towards the stomach. The wall of the stomach is made up of three thick layers of muscle. One layer is composed of longitudinal, one of circular, and the other of diagonal fibers. The powerful contractions of these muscles break up the food, mix it with gastric juices, and move it down the tract. Gastric juice is a mixture of hydrochloric acid and enzymes that further digests the food. The small gastric glands in the lining of the stomach secrete gastric juice and mucus. The mucus helps protect the stomach from its own digestive enzymes and acid. Partially digested food is pushed into the small intestine. Within the small intestine bile from the liver, that has been stored in the gallbladder, is mixed with pancreatic juices from the pancreas. The secretions of the pancreas contain enzymes that complete the digestive process. The connection between the absorption of glucose and amino acids as in the enzymatic digestive process is as follows: when glucose and/or free amino acids approach the cell membrane they are bound by special groups of enzymes that are within the membrane. The nutrients are then transported across the intestinal epithelium into the blood. Proteases are enzymes that hydrolyze proteins, which are long chains of amino acids joined together by a peptide bond. Like pepsin of the stomach theses enzymes will only break the peptide bonds between certain amino acids. 50% of body weight is composed of amino acid. In each region of the digestive tract rhythmic like waves of constrictions move the food down the tract. This form of contractile activity is called peristalsis and involves the involuntary smooth muscles. There are two layers of smooth muscles throughout most of the digestive tract.

Source, type, and action of digestive enzymes
Pancreas-chymotrypsin-digests proteins
Pancreas-proteases-hydrolyzes proteins
Pancreas-lipase-digests lipids
Saliva-amylase-acid of the stomach inhibits actions resulting in no starch metabolized
It also may hydrolyze starch to maltose
Saliva-ptyalin-acts the same as amylase
Body cells-nuclease-catalyzes the hydrolysis of nucleic acid
Raw food-cellulose-breaks down the fiber in the food
Stomach-rennin-coagulates milk protein making them ready for an enzyme attack
Stomach-pepsin-splits long proteins into shorter fragments (peptides)

Metabolism

Metabolism is the sum of the physical and chemical processes in an organism by which its material substance is produced, maintained, and/or destroyed. It is a process by which energy is made available. The process involves the expenditure of minimal energy for the maintenance of the respiratory, circulatory, peristalsis, muscle tones, body temperature, glandular activity and other vegetative function of the body. There is one chemical process that is associated with metabolism that may cause medical problems on its own. This process is metabolic acidosis which is caused by the interference with the normal metabolic process and/or from the production of lactic acidosis. This results in acid production. If at the same time, as the above takes place, the kidney fails to secrete sufficient NH4 it may cause ammonalysis, where the H2O is replaced by NH2.

Pancreas

The pancreas gland secrets digestive fluids into a person's intestines. It also secretes insulin that helps to promote the entry into the cells of glucose, fatty acids, and amino acids. It promotes glycogen protein, and lipid synthesis, and inhibits protein degradation, and lipolysis.(the decomposition of fat) Within these pancreatic digestive fluids are the enzymes amylase, trypsin, and lipid. The key enzyme in this process is the amylase enzyme that breaks down the starch, within the digestive process. It catalyzes the hydrolysis of starch into saccharine, maltase, or glucose. The trypsin enzyme converts the protein, as in red meat, into peptone. Peptone is a class of diffusible, soluble, substance, into which the proteins are converted, by partial hydrolysis, within the digestive tract. In this hydrolysis process the compound involved is split into fragments, by the addition of H2O, with the hydroxyl group being incorporated in one fragment, and the hydrogen atom in the other. As a result of the above processes, acid and alkaline juices are secreted simultaneously in response to the incoming protein in the red meat and the incoming starch. The protein and the starch promptly neutralize one another and leave a weak, watery solution in the stomach. This solution digests neither the protein and/or the starch properly. As a result the protein putrefies, and the starch ferments, as a result of the constant presence of bacteria in the digestive tract. As a result putrefaction and fermentation causes digestive problems. The bloodstream picks up the toxins from the putrefied fermented mess sending reversible toxic protein through out the body causing damage to body's cells and tissues..

Jehovah said to Moses"I have heard the murmurs of the children of Israel" "Tell them to eat bread in the morning and flesh at night". What he was referring to, regarding body processes, was that the pancreas secrets two enzymes, one for the protein in red meat, and one for starch. If a person eats too much starch, with the protein in the red meat, the protein in the red meat may not be metabolized. It is the pancreas's exocrine part, consisting of the secretor units (pancreatic acine) that produce and secrets into the duodenum a pancreatic juice which contains enzymes essential to protein digestion. The unmetabolized protein is called an inflammatory reversible toxic protein (cytokine) that results in an auto immune reaction. This auto immune reaction, involving the cyctokine, attacks the body's cells including the breast cells changing the protoplasm of the cell, exclusive of the cell nucleus, but involving most of the chemical activity of the cell. The results are the possible division (cytokine sis) and/or the degeneration of the cell.

Phosphorylation/dephosphorylation

In 1953 Edwin Krebs and Edmund Fischer discovered the process called phosphorlation. They were awarded the Nobel Prize for this discovery in 1992. Unfortunately, to the best of my knowledge this very important discovery has resulted in no constructive data, relative to the body's health, being proposed by the medical establishment.

They discovered the mechanism that cells use to regulate a wide variety of metabolic processes. This mechanism is called phosphorylation, a protein, that at times may act as a reversible protein resulting in dephosphorylation. This protein acts on the internal workings that maintain life in all cells and in many of the ways in which cells cooperate in tissues and organs. They discovered that if a phosphate molecule was attached to an inactive form, at a key location, the enzyme suddenly becomes active. They also showed that if a phosphate was removed by another enzyme that the first enzyme lapsed into inactivity. The enzyme that leads to phosphorylation are called protein kinases (transfers the enzyme). Dephosphorylation is the removal of a phosphate group from an organic compound as in the changing of ATP to ADP! * Phosphorylase is an enzyme that is contained in animal and plant tissue and that in the presence of an inorganic phosphate catalyzes the conversion of glycogen into sugar! Glycogen is similar to starch and constitutes the principle carbohydrate storage material in animals. It occurs chiefly in the liver, in musk, in fungi, and yeast! (it is called animal starch)

After reviewing the above it is possible to visualize how any auto immune reaction, affecting the body's key enzymes, could mean the destruction of the body's cells with cancer possible. In this case the key enzyme affected by the autoimmune process, in conjunction with the above, is the enzyme produced by the pancreas that is responsible for metabolizing the protein in the red meat.

Adenosine triphospate ATP is a nucleotide of several phosphate esters of nuceosides which is the basic unit of nucleic acid that functions as coenzymes that are vital to the energy process of all living cells.

Adenosine d phosphate ADP is a nucleotide vital to the energy process of all living cells during biological oxidation.

Energy is stored in the ATP molecule as ADP is converted to ATP which later converts back to ADP releasing the energy needed for muscular contractions

Genetics

Genes contain all the information that the body requests for the synthesis of a product. Each gene has a specific position on the chromosome map, from the stand point of function. Some of the key genes related to the body processes are: Immune Response that governs the immune response to certain antigens. Immune Suppressor that governs the ability of suppressing T cells in order to respond to certain antigens. Lethal, that the presence of which, brings about the death of an organism and/or permits its survival, but only under certain conditions. Regulation, whose product affects the activity of other genes,. Repressor, that doesn't always function to produce the maximum number of enzymes. Supplementary, are two independent pairs of genes which interact in such a way that either one may dominate and produce its own effect despite the absence of the other. I believe that the reason why genetics is one of the key body processes is that the secretions of the digestive enzymes are regulated by two factors neural and hormonal. Neural control is usually based on the body sensing a physical mass of food. This stimulation generally results from a stretching of the digestive tract. Meanwhile, the salivary, and some gastric enzymes secretions, are stimulated by smelling, tasting, and even thinking about food. Hormonal control is more specific. The presence of specific kinds of molecules, in the ingested foods themselves, stimulates receptor cells to produce a specific hormone. The hormone circulates in the blood until it reaches the secreting organ which it controls. The above process, less digestive enzymes, means medical problems. The best example of the genetic process is this writer's problems with lactose. As a result of a genetic defect, I lack the enzyme, lactase, which is necessary to catalyze lactose. As a result, if I ingest any lactose there's a build up of lactic acid within the blood. In turn, I develop a metabolic acidosis disease. This disease is caused by the interference with the intermediating metabolism and/or from the production of lactic acidosis, otherwise knows as excess lactic acid, within the blood. At the same time, the kidney may fail to secrete sufficient ammonia (NH4). This leads to ammonification, which in turn produces a fungus called aspergillum. In this writer's case it resulted in the formation of auriculars, a fungus covering the external parts of the ears. Lactose is one of the so-called inactive agents within some drugs that in some people may cause the drug to fail to properly metabolize.

Peristalsis process

The peristalsis process, within the body, assists the body's autonomic process in moving food through the body. It also assists the autonomic process in moving urine through the urethra and solid waste through the alimentary canal. It acts by creating waves of contractions and revelations of the tubular muscular system, especially the alimentary canal. Assisting the above is fiber, a filamentous matter, which is obtained from the structural and the bast tissue of plants, including leafy vegetables. It consists of carbohydrates, such as cellulose and/or pectin, and in particular the amorphous colloidal carbohydrate, that occurs in fruits, especially apples. The fiber the structural part of plants consists of carbohydrates, as cellulose and pectin, that are wholly or partially indigestible and when eaten stimulate the peristalsis process in the intestine. The fruits should be eaten on an empty stomach since they go directly to the lower intestine. The use of hot foods and/or drinks may restrict the peristalsis process.

Excretory/elimination process

All of the body's excretory processes involve the body's autonomic process. The excretory process is made up of four different functions. **Insensible perspiration**, which is a loss of fluid, from the body, by evaporation that normally occurs during breathing, with the main agent excreted carbon dioxide. **Sweat perspiration** which is a loss of about 10% of the body's waste fluids, from a reaction to heat and/or exercise, and is made up of water, salt (sodium chloride), phosphate, urea, ammonia, and other waste products. **Urinary Waste**, which is an autonomic process and is composed of water, urea, sodium, potassium chloride, phosphates, uric acid, organic salts and pigment. The urine is secreted by the kidney, transported by the urethra to the bladder, where it is stored in the bladder, and voided through the urethra. **Feces Waste** is primarily solid waste, from the digestive tract. It contains water, food remains, bacteria, and fluids, from the intestines, and the liver. It is formed in the intestines, and released via the rectum. The solid waste is assisted in its removal, from the body, by the peristalsis process within the body's autonomic process. This process creates waves of contractions and relaxations of the tubular muscular system, especially the alimentary canal by which its contents are forced through the system. This writer found that I have normal timely bowel movements if I assist the peristalsis process by ingesting apples and apple cider juice, on a daily basis. The apple products contain cellulose and/or pectin that assist in the activation of the peristalsis process. By assisting the body's peristalsis process, along with chewing my food completely, I always found that I had a normal, timely, bowel movement, between 5 am., the time I awake, and 6 am. The stool is always odorless, light colored, soft, and complete.

EFFECTS OF INGESTED POLLUTANTS

In order to fully understand the significance of ingesting a pollutant, within the overall equation, it is necessary to differentiate a medical problem, from ingesting a virus and/or bacteria, to one from ingesting a pollutant. If this is not accomplished, an adverse autoimmune reaction, to an ingested pollutant, may be treated as a bacterial infection etc., which may lead to the wrong use of medications.

When one looks at ingested pollutants, in relationship to the body's mental and physical well being, it is a fact that the world has more pollution within the air, drink, food, and medications, than was prevalent 20 years ago. Recently, it was reported that ten million people are at risk for lung infections, cancers, and shorted life expectancy, because they live in the ten worst polluted cities in the world. Three Russian cities are among the most polluted: Dzherzhinsk, Norilsk, and Rudnaya Pristan. The others are Linfen, China; Haina, Dominican Republic; Ranipet, India; Mayluu-Suu, Kyrgyzstan; La Oroya, Peru; Chernobyl, Ukraine; and Kabwe, Zambia. China is the most polluted country in the world. Also, as a result of air tight homes, with their various chemicals, indoor air has become 8 times worse than outdoor air. It has been reported that there are more greenhouse gases, carbon dioxides, in the atmosphere today than at any point during the past several hundred years. In Chicago, they were able to find that infants, in households where people smoked, are more than twice as likely to die of sudden infant death syndrome, as those in a smoke free environment. It was reported that seven people moved out of the sealed spacecraft lab, after only a six month stay, because of rising levels of atmospheric carbon dioxide. The Russians had to abandon a space craft because of high levels of mold/fungus. In California, there has been a 270% increase in autism caused by the carbon monoxide pollution, in the air, that is ingested by pregnant women. California air is cleaner now, but troubles remain. This writer in the mid 1950s was in California for a full summer and people were leaving California to escape the air pollution. In 1955, downtown Los Angeles experienced the nation's worst ever prolonged ozone pol-

38

lution: in one day. The hourly average levels of choking ozone were six times the maximum allowable rate under current federal standards. A report out of the University of California indicated that a study of infant deaths, within the Los Angeles County region, found that smog may be linked to infant deaths. Just recently California air regulators unanimously approved the world's most stringent rules to reduce auto emissions, that are said to contribute to global warming.

Recently, I was in China with a tour group, when I entered my hotel room, in Beijing; I had an immediate reaction to passive smoke and had to have my room changed. My new room was on the top floor overlooking the country side that contained a beautiful mountain. Unfortunately, while I was in Beijing for four sunny days I could only see this mountain one day because of the air pollution. It was obvious where the air pollution was coming from, when I observed nothing but bumper to bumper traffic all day long. One member of the tour group was from California and she experienced the same problems, as this writer, with her initial hotel room. When I commented to her about the air pollution, she mentioned that it reminded her of Los Angeles a few years ago. It was found that the risks of heart attacks increase on days of exposure to high air pollution.

This writer first came in contact with ingested pollutants while working in a production plant that used polyurethane foam in the production of soft drink machines. One day one of the workers accidentally mixed two chemical, involving the polyurethane foam, together, within the mixing machine. That night with the shop shut up tight, the maintenance man and this writer proceeded to clean the machines. Both the maintenance man and this writer developed severe breathing problems. The maintenance man, who was a heavy smoker, died of emphysema within six months. This writer from this point on developed adverse reactions to agents' and substances that had never affected me before. The key chemical involved, in the polyurethane foam, was isocyanides which was part of Germany's poison gas during World War II.

As you review the data on ingested pollutants keep in mind that, at times, it is not only the pollutant itself that may trigger an adverse reaction, but the quantity of the ingested pollutant. While this writer has had many personal problems with ingested pollutants, I believe my experience with preservatives stands out! I had a salad with all fresh vegetables yet developed an adverse auto immune reaction. The problem was in the pickles, that were in vinegar, and that you were told to refrigerate after opening. The pickles contained the strongest preservative on the market, titanium dioxide.. When I contacted the product manager, of a well know pickle manufacturer, and asked him why the strongest preservatives on the market was in the pickles, he informed me it was to maintain the color. Another example, was my experience with preservatives in a potato salad. The media article was titled, BACTERIA PROMPTS a RECALL OF POTATO SALAD SOLD IN New England. The article went on to say that they suspected that the salad might contain listeria monocytogenes bacteria that could cause serious and sometimes fatal infections. Four years to the day that this article appeared in the media I went into the same market that had issued the recall and purchased some prepackaged potato salad. When a friend and this writer ate this potato salad this writer and my friend had an adverse auto immune reaction. Ironically, this friend normally would not react to ingested agents that this writer would react to. However, in this case both my friend and this writer had an adverse auto immune reaction. The reason for our problems was that, usually, this type of product would have one very strong preservative in it, however; in this case the product had two strong preservatives. It was obvious that the potato salad manufacture, in an attempt to prevent any further costly recalls, put a second strong preservative in the potato salad. While the FDA has guide lines for the amount of any specific preservative that may be used in a particular substance they have no guide lines for the total number of preservatives that may be in a particular substance. Naturally, there are other pollutants in foods that may cause problems. Possibly the real shocker for this writer was the findings regarding cereal. In the article it indicated that the chemical acrylamide, in the cereal, coupled with eating other foods with acrylamide in it, may cause a person medical problems. The article went on to say that acrylamide forms during traditional cooking methods, whether from ready made foods or from raw ingredients, fried or baked, in a home kitchen. It forms when a naturally occurring amino acid called asparagine is heated to very high temperatures with certain sugars such as glucose. Potatoes are especially rich in both asparagines and glucose and thus produce lots of acrylamide especially in potato chips. The major food products that cause adverse autoimmune reactions are peanuts, eggs, milk, tree nuts, soybeans, and shell fish. From a personal experience I had an adverse autoimmune reaction to various agents and or substances

Auto immune triggers Gluten, in wheat products. <u>Colorants,</u> In food drink and drugs. <u>Nuts</u>, from the leguminous plant. Whey, in margarine. Ham, if it contains a soy product. <u>Protein,</u> in red meat. if it is unmetabolized. <u>Mold</u>, on the outer surface of vegetables such as cauliflower and broccoli. <u>Cheese</u>, cooked or uncooked. <u>Protein</u>, in cat saliva that is transferred to cat dander. <u>Chocolate</u>, from the seeds of the cacao plant that contains theobromine. <u>Carbon dioxide and Carbon monoxide. Starch</u>, if not metabolized. <u>Yeast</u>, a fungi if transformed into a mycelia (mold) stage under certain environmental conditions. <u>Fungus</u>, a parasitic plant that lacks chlorophyll. There are 110 different strains of fungus that causes human medical problems. Dicotyledonous plant family, which is. a two cotyledon cup like hollow plant that includes grapes. Leguminous plant family,. which is a pod or seed vessel type plant that includes soy and nuts. Acrylamide, an acrylic amide chemical that is created in foods when starches and other carbohydrates are overheated during cooking, particularly fried foods. Acrylamide, may be carcinogenic to some humans. Shell fish and previously frozen fish. Fish, causes the most adverse reactions among people. Lactose, which is usually a genetic problem wherein the body lacks an enzyme that metabolizes the lactose. Preservatives, particularly those that contain metals, such as sodium and titanium dioxide. It is not only the specific preservative that may cause the adverse reaction, but the quantity of that preservative. The FDA has strict guide lines on the amount of any specific preservative within a product, but no guide lines as to the total amount of all preservatives within a given product. I had a friend that normally did not have an adverse reaction to preservatives. However, when a prepackaged potato salad contained two strong preservatives both my friend and this writer had severe adverse reactions. The supplier had put in the two strong preservatives rather than the usual one preservative in an attempt to prevent a previous problem with e coli bacteria, resulting in a recall of the potato salad.

In association with the above one must take care when taking medicine and certain foods. For example, calcium in milk impairs the absorption of tetracycline. MAO inhibitors react badly with the tyraminein in foods such as aged cheese, chicken livers, sausages, and wine. Also, one should be concerned about the risks of mixing drugs and herbs. For example St. John's Wort, which is used for depression, is one of the most studied herbs. It appears to speed up the pace at which the body metabolizes drugs, diluting their effects. The Mayo Clinic in Rochester, Minn. reported that we barely know what one herb does on its own, let alone what might take place when you mix it in four or five prescription drugs. Possibly, the real shocker to this writer, involving food and medications, came in a media article by Dr. G.. In the article he said that if he listed all the medications that adversely react with grapefruit juice it would fill his column for the next week or more.

Pollutants in the air

Fungus/mold is a major air pollutant. The key fungi that include members of the genera are aspergillus, penicillium, and cladesporiu. A mold is a downy or furry growth on the surface of organic matter caused by fungi, especially in the presence of dampness or decay. A fungus is any of a large division (eumycota) of thallophytes including molds, mildew, mushrooms, rusts, and smuts, which are parasites on living organisms or feed upon dead organic material. They reproduce by means of spores! There are 10,000 species of fungi with about 10 causing illnesses. Early one morning while entering a super market along side a little girl with her Mother I overheard the little girl tell her Mother that she felt sick. The Mother said to her, every time we come in here you get sick let's get out of here. Based on my own experience her sickness had to be caused by the fungus/mold in the dairy section, which was right opposite the door, we entered. Some people have labeled this reaction the grocery store syndrome since it so common. Also, at the very opposite end of the super market, while standing along side a baker, from the bakery, I had an adverse reaction to the yeast used in the bakery. This is called crossover where the body's immune system can't tell the difference between the good yeast, a fungi, and the bad fungus in the dairy section. Fungus was found on the wall of a brand new condo in Florida! With the high humidity that leads to the growth of fungus in Florida one must control the humidity from the very beginning. It means air-conditioning seven days per week twenty four hours per day. A Tottenville New York library had to close because of poisonous fungus growth on the basement walls. The Hilton hotel chain sued a contractor for mold infestation in a brand new hotel in Honolulu. This writer and two friends were in the Nashua public library and it became very warm so they turned on the air-conditioning. This writer and one of my friends had a reaction to the fungus blowing out of the air ducts. At an aging senior center the thrift shop was shut down between 12 o'clock and 1 o'clock. When they opened the door at one o'clock the odor from the fungus caused some people in the adjoining room to become sick.

Carbon monoxide CO is another major air pollutant. It is a serious ingested pollutant because it deprives the body of oxygen and may be fatal to some people. The dangers of CO poisoning occurs more often in winter. The risk of CO poisoning is greatest in the winter months because of decreased ventilation and better insulation within the homes, along with the increase use of the heating systems. CO is also very hazardous for children because they have a tendency to be enclosed in vehicles, with the windows up tight, with the engine running. One of the more serious reactions to CO involved the refuse driver. One morning his wife had trouble awakening him for work and ended up calling 911. The Doctors said that if they had arrived just two hours later he would have died before they could help him. The problem was CO with a severe loss of oxygen. This particular refuse driver was responsible for making the actual pick up of the refuse as well as moving the truck from stop to stop. In order to speed up the process he left the engine running. Unfortunately, the big truck exhaust pipe was pointed at the cab's side window that was open, filling the truck cab with Carbon monoxide. The media article said that the EPA office was going to screen their own office following birth defects among their employees. One visit by this writer to the EPA building and it was obvious what the problem was. The EPA building had an unventilated underground garage. It also had two large elevators that went from the upper floors down to the underground garage. The CO went right up the elevators with the employees ingesting it on the way up and they continued to ingest the CO as they sat at their desks

Combination of carbon monoxide and fungus. Most people when they think about indoor pollution they think of the slums and/or the tenement buildings. However, the ultimate example of indoor pollution is at the White House. People who visit the White House never want to go back since they found it moldy and murky. The White House pollution is a combination of fungus from the aged building and CO from the enclosed underground garage. There is a $300 million renovation of the White House to clean up the pollution and improve security against weapons of mass destruction. At the same time as these renovations are being made to protect the occupants of the White House some of the occupants are experiencing some medical problems from pollutants in the White House.

The various medical problems related to ingesting pollutants in the White House by some of its occupants are as follows: Reagan, first of all spent more time living in the White House than any other modern President. His apparent predisposition towards Alzheimer's disease and the long term ingesting of White House pollutants contributed to his Alzheimer's disease. Ford was diagnosed with Actinomycosis and had symptoms similar to many autoimmune reactions especially a swollen tongue. As a matter of fact, the doctors extended his hospital stay as doctors tried to figure out what was causing his painful and swollen tongue. Actinomycosis is an infection caused by inhaling of Actinomyces Israelli, which is a bacteria/fungus agent, which easily could have originated within the White House pollution. Bush senior, his wife, and even his dog, were reported by a doctor at the Queens Medical Center in Nottingham England as suffering from graves disease. Graves's disease is caused by an environmental agent, which causes an adverse autoimmune reaction that attacks the body, particularly the thyroid gland. Once again this ties in with White House pollution. James Carter, while not having any medical problems, that may be directly connected to the White House pollution, had a medical condition that was aggravated by the White House pollution. This medical condition was hemorrhoids. At one time he had to leave a Christmas party in the White House for staffers to receive emergency treatment for his painful hemorrhoids. At times he was unable to participate in any kind of public events because he was incapacitated from his hemorrhoids. Clinton of all the occupants of the White House within this writer's knowledge personified the problems that Americans have with ingested pollutants. Ironically Clinton could not escape from ingesting pollutants since his only homes for many years were the polluted Arkansas and White House mansions. Also, Clinton was highly subjected to allergic/autoimmune reactions. Unfortunately, there is evidence that Clinton may have been incorrectly given medications for a disease and/or virus type infections when his medical problem was a reaction to ingesting pollutants both in the White House and outside the White House. As a result in at least one case he had an inflammation of the inner ear canal and the drugs he took damaged the hearing organ causing a loss of hearing. Maybe it is catchy among White House occupants since President Bush similar to President Carter had hemorrhoids. However, the direct tie in with White House pollution was Bush's fainting experience. It was reported that bush felt faint, while sitting down eating pretzels, while watching TV. From the facts reported this writer conclude that Bush was acting normal by watching TV while eating pretzels and similar to many other people he over ate. His fainting type condition was caused by the yeast in the pretzels. He experienced an autoimmune reaction called vertigo which was caused by the body's reaction to the yeast, a fungi, and the fungus in the polluted White House. The process is called cross over, with the body's autoimmune process unable to tell the difference between the good yeast, a fungi, and the bad fungus and as a result reacts to both with the same intensity.

Hair pollutants Finally, a less technical source of pollutants, but at times just as serious, are the pollutants primarily carbon monoxide one carries on their clothing and in their hair. In the case of the hair the pollutant may be transferred to the pillow case with possible medical problems from the inhalation of the pollutants during the sleep cycle from either the hair and/or the pillowcase.

CAUSE AND PREVENTION OF MEDICAL PROBLEMS

While I have documented data on the cause and prevention of more serious medical problems I selected the EAR to start off this chapter for several reasons. First, it was not only the first medical problem that I encountered it also proved to be the start of my accumulating documented data on several medical problems, some serious. Also, at the same time I accumulated data on the poor quality of our health care. At that time, I did not have an appreciation for the requirement of the need for the average person to help themselves, in addressing medical problems, to assist them to a healthier life. The ear infection problem reflected all the factors that the average person had to address. These factors, involving medical problems, were the wrong diagnosis, wrong medication, and the wrong dosage. However, above all it demonstrated that the Medical Scientific Establishment and Associated Foundations (MSE&AF) failed to properly understand and/or properly address the key body processes that served as the basis of so many chronic diseases, the body's auto immune process.

Ears

It all started when I was temporarily helping a friend take care of his two year old daughter, while his wife was in the hospital having a baby. One day, I had this young girl out to the park playing happily, with her only concern being when was she going to have her lunch, and when was she going to have her nap. That evening, her father announced that he was taking her to see the pediatrician. I naturally assumed it was for a check up, since the father never mentioned any medical problems. When they came home, from the pediatrician, the father had a medical prescription, for 500mg of amoxicillin, for his daughter. The father asked this writer if I would get the prescription filled, the following day, and get his daughter started on the prescription. Despite my lack of knowledge about medical prescriptions, since while I growing up there were few drugs available, and what drugs were available were too expensive for my poor family, I was very concerned about an obviously high dosage of this drug. When I went to the pharmacist to have the prescription filled I voiced my concerns, to him, about such an apparent large dosage for a two year old. While I could tell that he was concerned, he naturally filled the prescription so that he would get the doctor in trouble.. When the father came home from work, I mentioned, to him, that I was very concerned about giving his daughter 500mg of amoxicillin. I mentioned to the father that as a child I had many severe ear aches with lots of pain. I pointed out that his daughter could not possibly have a real ear infection since she had no pain. Fortunately, he decided not to give his daughter this drug.

Shortly after the above incident, an article appeared in the paper that caught my eye. The article stated that ear infection rates are soaring among children. The article went on to say that office visits to the doctor, for ear infections, among children under 2 years, have soared to 224%. In the article it claimed that leading specialists are questioning this big increase. Some specialists blamed it on the fact that more children were using day care services. The next media article that caught this writer's eye stated that doctors don't always get ear infections right. The article went on to say that when parents bring their children, to the doctor, who in turn diagnoses the child with an ear infection, it is automatic antibiotics. The article went on to say that the pediatrician probably can't make the correct diagnosis more than half the time. It also indicated that most of the drugs, given for ear infections, probably don't help anymore. The article stated that many pediatricians mistakenly prescribe more and more powerful antibiotics, for an ear infection, that don't seem to respond to the medication. The next media article of importance was titled, RISE IN INFANT HEARING LOSS PUZZELS EXPERTS. The article said, that medical experts, at three major hearing treatment centers, reported that the number of cases, of severe hearing loss, in infants, has dramatically increased in the last year. The doctors are concerned and puzzled about the cause. In none of the above media articles was there any mention of an autoimmune reaction and/or that it was not a true so called ear infection. The next article of significance was about, a former Miss America, who lost her, hearing after taking an anti biotic (gentamicin) for an ear infection when she was 18 months old. With the above documented data as background, I began to gather data on the so called ear infection problems. First, I found that what was thought to be an ear infection was not a true ear infection at all. I found that in most cases the so called ear infection was really a severely inflamed inner ear canal that gave all the appearances of an ear infection. This inflamed inner ear was generally caused by an adverse auto immune reaction from an ingested agent and/or substance which the body perceived as a foreign agent and/or substance. This writer believes that when the doctor saw this highly inflamed inner ear the doctor felt that they could not take any chances that it wouldn't turn into meningitis, so they medicated. In some cases, such as my friend's two year old, they medicated heavily. I called a leading amoxicillin manufacture and informed him that amoxicillin, once know as the golden drug for ear infections is now only 30% effective and I know why. When I told him that the reason why the drug is so ineffective is that it is not being used for a true ear infection, but for an adverse autoimmune reaction, his immediate response was, "you aren't going to alarm the public are you". I also informed him that some people have an adverse autoimmune reaction, which resembles an ear infection, from the preservatives within the amoxicillin itself. This preservative is the strongest preservative on the market, titanium dioxide. I also found that one amoxicillin manufacture doesn't recommend amoxicillin for any child two years or younger, and the dosage for children over 2 years of age is only 45mg. This writer found, that regardless, if you are a child and/or an adult, if you take any medications, particularly antibiotics, for a non ear type infections; it could cause at least one serious problem, a hearing loss. The medication damages and/or destroys the auditory nerve fibers, within the cochlear canal, within the inner ear. These hair cells initiate the impulses, via the fibers, of the auditory nerve to the brain. The end result is a hearing loss. President Clinton developed a hearing loss as a result of the above process

While the above took place in the 1990s, here it is 01-18-07, and the medical scientific establishment continues to miss the point. They don't understand the above processes and/or how to properly address them before the fact rather than after the fact. I believe that the AP media article, on 01-18-07, says it all. Toddler study casts doubt on ear tubes. Infections not tied to slower learning. Most toddlers with frequent ear infections don't need ear tubes to preserve normal learning, and behavior through primary school, according to a study challenging one big reason for these common procedures. Repeated ear infections, even some colds, can leave a fluid build up that specialists long feared would dampen hearing and slow language and other learning. However, it now appears the hearing loss is too short-lived and mild to interfere with learning, at least in the vast majority of children. In 2004, professional groups eased the guidelines that had long dictated quick surgery to clear accumulated fluid. The children in the study were tested for skills in hearing sounds, reading, writing, socializing, conduct, and intelligence. Children who got ear tubes quickly did no better than those who waited up to nine months for a check up to see whether the fluid remained, and only then got implants if needed. Plastic tubes are implanted in the eardrums to ventilate the middle ear, cut down on future fluid, and drain it when infections develop. There are no reliable current estimates on how many ear tubes are implanted each year. About 550,000 were placed in 1996, with about half in toddlers. It has been the number two surgery in the nation, after circumcision.

New England fungus

While fungus is not an unique medical problem to only New England I have attached the fungus label to New England as a result of the media article titled NEW ENGLANDERS ON THE DEATH OF THEIR HEALTH CARE, along with the associated factors contained within the media article in support of the headline. The article went on to say that New England has more of its work force than any other part of the United States engaged in health care, with more treatments. New England states are not free of spiraling Medicare costs. If New Englanders require hospital treatment some of the best health care professionals are located in NE. NE residents are not healthier than other parts of the US. Also, despite the fact that New Englander's eat a little less and exercise a little more than other parts of the US. they are not healthier. NE is plagued with soaring medical costs with mediocre health results

More significant is the fact that the NE. Fungus is the precursor to more serious medical problems. NE. leads the nation in incidents of breast cancer, asthma, and chronic medical problems. While it might be said that NE. Fungus might be indirectly tied into breast cancer the same can not be said about asthma and chronic medical problems. In particular, the auto immune reaction to the Fungus ties in with the fact that the body's auto immune process is directly related to the majority of chronic medical problems. It has been reported that in all of New England the Cape has the greatest number of medical problems. I believe that this may be as a result of it's location with the ocean on both sides. As a result, this location it lends itself to ongoing problems with fog and/or mist that lends itself to mold/fungus. Added to the above is the carbon monoxide pollution from the auto traffic jams.

Prior to providing specific data on the cause and prevention of the New England Fungus medical problem I believe the reader should be informed about the facts involving Fungi. There are 10,000 species of Fungi with 10 causing serious medical problems. It is important to note that the Fungus lives by decomposing and absorbing the organic material in which they grow. Fungus is any of a large division of thallophytes, including molds, mildew, mushrooms, rusts, and smuts, which are parasites on living organisms or feed upon dead organic material. They reproduce by means of spores in the presence of dampness or decay.

Some cause spoilage of foodstuffs and deterioration of leather goods, paper, fabrics, and lumber.

Also, I believe that the reader should be interested in the fact that while fungus is more prevalent in the slums it is found in other segments of society. They found Fungus in an orbiting space craft. The White House was loaded with Fungus. People who visited the White House refused to go back since they found it moldy and murky. At the present time the White House is going through a $300 million renovation to clean up the pollutants and make it more secure. This writer while visiting a brand new condo complex in Florida became ill from the fungus in the stuffed chair. Also, within the same condo complex they found Fungus on the wall of a new unoccupied condo.

What is unique about NE Fungus is that its source is unlike any other parts of the country. The source of the growth of Fungus, in NE., is the age of the buildings, and the old style of the buildings. Usually the buildings were built with a cellar, not a basement, and an attic. Both areas are ideal for the development of dampness and moisture necessary for the growth of Fungi. Usually these sections of the buildings have no vents blowers etc: to release any pollutants. Added to the above is the change in life style of the building residents. Today the residents spend more time indoors with their TVs and computers. Also, as a result of the increased crime rate the buildings are locked up tight with no vents etc:. Two examples of the above are the Federal EPA office in downtown Boston, and the 175 year old Boston church. The EPA office is located in a very old building in downtown Boston. It has an underground, under the building, garage with no vents openings etc:. It has an elevator that goes from the garage up to the upper floors containing the offices. There are no stairs. The Fungus and the carbon monoxide vapors never leave the garage and join the EPA employees as they go up the elevator to their desks. The media reported that many employees became very sick and many employees experienced birth defects among their children. The 175 year old church found that they had Fungus everywhere and found that despite all attempts to clean up the Fungus they could not get rid of it. One doesn't have a chance in NE. it may be fungus where you work, fungus at home and fungus in your church.

While the body's reaction to the Fungus is the source of the medical problems plaguing NE. unfortunately, the medical profession is not addressing the reactions involved. The body's auto immune reaction to the Fungus is not properly understood and/or properly addressed by the medical profession. As a result, the process leads to the wrong use of medications, and/or the over use of medications, which results in contracting chronic medical problems. Medications only compound the problem since the only solution to the NE. medical problems is the elimination of the Fungus pollutant.

Compounding the above is that most people who have an autoimmune reaction to the Fungus also have an auto immune reaction to yeast. It is called cross-over wherein the body's auto immune process can't tell the difference between the good yeast, a fungi, and the bad Fungus and reacts adversely to both. On a personal basis I had this problem when I ate a large amount of cookies with yeast in them. If I did not go to my knees I would have fallen. President Bush had this problem when he ate a lot of pretzels with yeast in them. It was reported that he fainted which is an adjunct to the usual adverse reaction of vertigo. Once again if the medical profession doesn't properly address this problem and attempts to medicate it could create serious medical problems from a combination of Fungus and yeast.

Bleach is the only sure chemical to remove fungus

World wide acrylamide

In the past I have had an adverse reaction to potato chips. However, at times I just have a taste for potato chips. Recently, I purchased some potato chips and as in the past I started out eating very small amounts. Unfortunately, I weakened and ate two large helpings of the chips. That evening I had three common adverse auto immune reactions. I had dry itchy eyes and dry itchy skin. However it was the third reaction that caused me the biggest problem. I had a full blown case of an inflamed bladder reducing the capacity of my bladder to hold urine. As in the past I had to get up several times throughout the night to urinate. I finally decided to attempt to find documented data on the agent that was triggering my body's adverse auto immune reaction. I found that the agent was a chemical called acrylamide an acrylic amide. Acrylamide is created in foods when the starches and other carbohydrates are overheated during cooking. Naturally, this chemical is prevalent in fried foods. What was really shocking is that acrylamide may be a carcinogenic to some humans.

I have used the term world wide to identify this medical problem since it is a key factor leading to the death of health care through out the world.

Attention deficit disorder (ADD)

The child is distracted as a result of their ongoing concerns about their body's adverse physical problems. As a result of this distraction, the child has trouble concentrating on anything else other than these physical problems. The key adverse physical problems are pressure on the bladder, with the need to urinate frequently, and pressure on the bowel, with a constant feeling on the part of the child to have a bowel movement. While the above physical problems may be alleviated there is one adverse physical problem that is not only ongoing, but is not relievable by the child. This physical problem is pressure on the inner ear, with all the symptoms of an ear infection, with the inflammation, but no pain. Also, many times vertigo is experienced by the child. To prevent ADD all agents and/ or substances within the child's diet, causing an adverse auto immune reaction, must be eliminated.

Vertigo

Vertigo is a dizziness type sensation of the body tilting within a stable surrounding. It is a type of an illusory sense that either the environment and/or one's own body is revolving. The above is caused by the displacement of the perilympa, a clear fluid within the inner ear canals. This fluid undisturbed allows for the body to maintain its balance. The displacement of the perilympa fluid is caused by the inflammation of the inner ear canals. Since this fluid is incompressible, the inflammation of the membrane causes the displacement of the perilympa fluid from the vestibular canal to the tympanic canal, resulting in vertigo. The inflammation of the inner ear canals is caused by an adverse auto immune reaction. The adverse reaction is caused by the body ingesting an agent and/or substance that the body considers to be foreign. For an example of how the process works I cite the grocery store incident, which some people call the grocery store syndrome. One day while going into the grocery store, just as it opened, I was joined by a young girl and her Mother. Immediately, upon entering the store the young girl complained to her Mother that she felt sick. The Mother said every time we come in here you get sick let's get out of here. The door that we entered was right opposite the dairy section. Based on this writer's personal experience, the girl had a reaction to the mold/fungus within the dairy section. While at this time I did not experience any severe vertigo, I did feel the beginning of a vertigo reaction. Ironically, on the same day I stopped to talk to the baker, on the opposite side of the store. At that time, I developed a strong vertigo reaction from the yeast on the bakers clothing. The process involved is called crossover, where the body's autoimmune process can not detect the difference between the bad fungus and the good yeast, which is a fungi, and reacts to both. Sometimes it is not only the agent itself but the quantity that may cause an autoimmune reaction. For example: I thought it was a good idea to eat some sweets to bring up my blood sugar content, prior to my daily walk. One day I ingested a large amount of cookies and had such a serious vertigo reaction, to the yeast in the cookies, that if I had not kneeled down, immediately, I would have fallen down.

Breast cancer

Prior to providing this writer's details on the possible cause and prevention of breast cancer I would like to provide the reader with two examples, of poor medical research, on the cause and prevention of breast cancer. The first is a quotation in a women's magazine by a woman doctor with the National Institute of Health and the wife of a US Congressman. ("I am really disturbed by my colleagues, recently, a close friend of mine died of breast cancer and the approach and treatment on her was identical to that of my Mother who died of the same breast cancer 20 years ago"). The second example involves this writer. I spent one whole week contacting several breast cancer foundations and/or cancer societies with an offer. I offered to donate a large sum of money, to their organization, if they could provide me with the name of a person and/or persons that were doing research on the cause and prevention of breast cancer. No one could provide a single name.

Breast cancer is the most common cancer of women in America. The rate of breast cancer increases between 30 to 50 years of age and reaches a peak at age 65. Breast cancer is caused by a malignant tumor of the breast cells. This malignant tumor is as a result of the body's adverse autoimmune process. In this process, the protein cytokine, although not an antibody, acts like an antibody, when it is released into the blood stream when the body makes contact with an antigen. In particular, it is when the body ingests the protein in red meat and starch together. Acid and alkaline juices are secreted in response to the incoming protein and starch, promptly neutralizing one another, and leaving a weak, watery, solution, in the stomach, that digests neither the protein and/or the starch properly. Instead, the protein putrefies, and the starch ferments, as a result of the constant presence of bacteria in the digestive tract. The blood stream picks up the toxins, from the putrefied fermented mess, and sends the toxins through out the body, and in particular into the breasts red blood cells, causing damage to them and/or destruction of them. Another possible cause is inflammation, which in turn is as a result of an adverse autoimmune reaction and/or as a result of a morbid enlargement, a new growth, of tissue, in which multiplication of cells is uncontrollable and progressive. This malignant cell is prone to the invasion of other cells, especially tumorgenic cells, which are prone to malignant tumors. A Dr. Marshall, an Immunologist from the University of Texas Medical School has said that it is difficult to zero in on the cause and prevention of breast cancer, since there are 24 different pathways for the breast cancer tumor to form. The National Institute of Health has offered $100 million to anyone who can detail how genes run amok. As far as the NIH is concerned BC is caused by genes running amok. This writer found that, not only did the genes not run amok they performed within their prescribed processes. I found that genes occur in pairs and they structure and regulate the way the body's normal cells and tissues develop. Also, genes control the interaction of cells which unfortunately includes both the normal cells and the abnormal cells. The two genes involved in BC. are the immune response IR, and immune suppressor IS genes. The IR gene governs the immune response to certain antigens. Naturally, those people without this gene are non responders to antigens. The IS gene governs the ability of the body to suppress the T cell in response to certain antigens. At this point, to fully understand this process, one must review the body's autoimmune process. (see AUTOIMMUNE PROCESS defined in the section on Effects of Body Processes). As noted, the key is the cytotoxic T cell or killer cell. This toxic cell has a toxin or antibody that may have a specific toxic destructive action upon cells of special organs. In addition to the above, there is the immunoglobin process where a structured related to glycol protein functions as an antibody coded for by different genes. Also, possibly involved in the overall processes are cells that become active in response to certain stimulation, such as leukocytes, that are found in the blood, that are the body's cells that react in contact with an antigen. Compounding the above is the phosphorylation/dephosphorylation process. In this process phosphorylation, a protein, may act as a reversible protein, resulting in dephosphorylation. This protein acts adversely on the internal workings that maintain life in the breast cell. It was discovered that if a phosphate molecule was attached to an inactive form, at a key location, the enzyme suddenly becomes active. Also, if this phosphate was removed by another enzyme, the first enzyme may lapse into inactivity. The enzyme that leads to phosphorylation is called protein kinases.

Recently there were two media articles supporting the relationship of red meat and breast cancer. In a report by Reuters, it said that researchers found in a study of 90,000 women ages, 26 to 46, over an eight year period, that 714 women developed breast cancer. They found that women who ate red meat raised their risk of contracting breast cancer. In an Associated Press report, it reported that eating red meat may raise a woman's risk of a common type of breast cancer. They found that women who ate more than 1 1/2 servings of red meat, per day, were twice as likely to develop hormone related breast cancer, as those who ate fewer than three portions per week. Finally, if these two reports have not convince the reader of the relationship of red meat and breast cancer they should consider what Jehovah said to Moses. Jehovah said to Moses "I have heard the murmurs of the children of Israel". "Tell them to eat bread in the morning and flesh at night." This ties in with the failure of the pancreas to properly metabolize the protein in the red meat when eaten with starch.

Alcohol and breast cancer linked

The media article headline read moderate drinking of alcohol linked to breast cancer.. Researchers led by Dr. Arthur Klatsky of the Kaiser Permanente Medical Care Program in Oakland Calif., revealed their findings at a meeting of the European Cancer Organization in Barcelona. Previous studies have shown a link between alcohol consumption and breast cancer, but there have been conflicting messages about whether different kinds of alcohol were more dangerous than others. In this study American researchers found that all types of alcohol-wine, beer or liquor-add equally to the risk of developing breast cancer in women. Researchers found no difference in the risk of developing breast cancer among women who drank wine, beer, or liquor. Compared with light drinkers, those who had less than one drink a day, to women who had one or two drinks a day increased their risk of developing breast cancer by 10 percent. Women who had more than three drinks a day raised their risk by 30 percent. According to data published in the British Journal of Cancer in 2002, 4 percent of all breast cancers-about, 44,000cases a year in the United Kingdom, are due to alcohol consumption.

This writer found that the chemical process involving alcohol and breast cancer involves yeast. Alcohol is produced by yeast fermentation of certain carbohydrates. Yeast is a single cell fungi of the phylumascomycota that is reproduced by fission and/or budding. The daughter cells often remain attached and are capable of fermenting carbohydrates into alcohol and carbon dioxide. Several yeasts of genus saccharmyces are used in brewing alcohol. Also, alcohol may be made by brewing sugar with yeast. Regardless of the process, the one constant throughout the process is the yeast. The key process involved is the body's autoimmune process, compounded by the body's synergism process. The body's auto immune process is unable to detect the difference between the good fungi, yeast, and the bad fungus. As a result the body's auto immune process treats yeast as a foreign agent and reacts to the yeast by attacking the body including red blood cells of the breast, causing breast caner. My suggestion is that a person attempt to avoid yeast in other products to have a chance of avoiding breast cancer while drinking alcohol.

Common cancers

The World Cancer Research Fund and the American Institute for Cancer reported that excessive body fat and red meat are linked to an increase risk of common cancers. The report went on to say that 40% of all cancers are linked to food, lack of exercise, and body weight. A panel of 21 researchers compiled a 571 page report that listed the key factors that link certain personal habits to the risk of contracting a common cancer. The report indicated that "the evidence that high body fatness and also physical inactivity are causes of a number of cancers is particularly strong". The report went on to say that body fat was convincingly linked to six cancers. They were esophagus, pancreas, colon, kidney and endometrium. Also, the report went on to say that the linking of red meat (beef, pork, lamb and goat) to colorectal cancer was more convincing than it was a decade ago. The panel recommended that people avoid processed meats such as bacon, ham, sausage and lunch meat. The panel found convincing evidence linking alcoholic drinks to cancers of the mouth, pharynx, larynx, esophagus, as well as colorectal cancer in men and pre-and post menopause cancer in women. In the documented data on breast cancer I believe I have identified the process involve in alcohol and cancers.

I thought it was ironic that the panel mentioned almost all the cancers except breast cancer. As noted in my documented data on breast cancer I was able to directly trace the process that causes breast cancer. It ties in with the reference to red meat, as in the above.

Autoimmune diseases

(**Source** US. Dept. of Health and Human Services)

There are more than 80 autoimmune diseases, affecting some 50 million Americans; 75 percent of those are women. Some people don't even know they have an autoimmune disease, as the symptoms vary widely. Below find a few key autoimmune diseases and the body's reaction.

FIBROMYALGIA In this disease the immune system attacks the muscles, tendons and ligaments, causing pain and fatigue. More than 80 percent of those diagnosed are women.

GRAVES DISEASE This thyroid disorder, which affects 3 million individuals in the United States, is one of the most common autoimmune diseases. It can lead to weight loss, tremors, and high blood pressure. Women are seven times more likely to develop this condition

HASHIMOTO THROIDITIS This condition causes low levels of thyroid hormone, resulting in weight gain, sensitivity to cold and goiters. It is 50 times more common in women than men. **INFLAMMATORY BOWEL DISEASE** This condition actually describes two disorders of the small intestines; ulcerative colitis, and Crohn's disease. Symptoms of ulcerative colitis include bloody diarrhea, pain, urgent bowel movements, joint pains, and skin lesions. Symptoms of Crohn's disease include chronic diarrhea, low-grade fever, fatigue, weight loss, abdominal cramps, and pain around the navel, or on the right side of the abdomen, joint pain, and skin lesions. Both are more common in women than men.
LUPUS This disease, an inflammation of the connective tissues, but can afflict every organ in the body. Symptoms include a bright rash on the face, joint pain, unexplained fever, chest pain, during inhalation, and hair loss. It is nine times more common in women than men **MULTIPLE SCLEROSIS** This disease, of the central nervous system, usually appears between the ages of 20 and 40. Symptoms include numbness, tingling or paralysis of the limbs, impaired vision, and tremors. It affects twice as many women as men..
RHEUMATOID ARTHRITIS In this disease the immune system attacks and inflames the membranes around the joints, causing pain, swelling, and loss of strength. About 70% of the estimated 2.1 million Americans affected, in 2004, were women. **SCLERODERMA.** In this disease immune cells produce scar tissue in the skin, internal organs and small blood vessels. Symptoms include eyes and mouth dryness, pain in the fingers and toes, and muscle soreness. Although the disease affects three times more women than men over all, it affects 15 times more women, of childbearing age than men.

The above medical problems are all caused by an adverse autoimmune reaction to an ingested agent and or substance. While the adverse reactions may affect many liquid glands of the body, with no immediate obvious symptoms, there are several basic symptoms. These symptoms are: Itchy eyes, from the loss of oxygen, and the blockage of the tear duct glands. Pressure, on the inner ear, and/or vertigo, from the swelling of the inner ear canal, causing a displacement of fluids. Dry mouth, from a lack of saliva, caused by swollen saliva glands. Dry itchy skin, from the blockage of mucin, melania, and/or keratin. Loss of taste and/or smell, from the inflammation of the taste buds and/or olfactory nerves. A dry itchy vagina, from the loss of lubricants as a result of swollen bartholin glands. Urinary incontinence, from a swollen bladder, causing an under capacity bladder.

Simply put the solution to many auto immune diseases is to avoid ingesting agents and/or substances that trigger the body's auto immune process.

Cervical cancer in New Hampshire

I became familiar with cervical cancer in New Hampshire (NH) as a result of an article in the media, and the medical experience of a woman friend. The article indicated that (NH) was fourth in the nation in cervical cancer incidents and a staggering first in cervical cancer deaths in the nation. Prior to detailing the experiences of my woman friend, I believe it is important to describe cervical cancer. Cervical cancer, neck or cervix, is the inflammation of the cervix of the uterus. The cervical carcinoma may involve a genetic predisposition along with problems with chronic irritation from a trauma, infection, etc:. Once again, it was almost as if I purposely planned a medical event in order to prove a point. A woman friend became involved in what this writer called the NH cervical cancer syndrome. This woman, on or about 02-22-95, went to a Women Doctor, on the staff of a major Nashua NH. hospital with an apparent vaginal infection. On her first visit the Dr. reported that Ms. B had a heavy discharge, and a fishy odor, from the vagina, which she did not have! Ms. B was not informed of the above, but it was recorded on her medical records. The so-called heavy discharge, with the fishy odor, came right out of the drug manual. During this visit, the Dr. indicated that Ms. B's vaginal problem was caused by a gardnerella G bacterium, but not a trichomonas (T) bacterium. On this first visit, the Dr. gave Ms. B a prescription for 4 capsules of 250 milligrams, of metronidazole (M), taken at the same time! The manufacture recommends this dosage for T only! Per the Mayo Lab G bacteria is not hard to identify, it is a rod shaped 0.5" in dia. and 1.5 to 2.5" in length! On or about 03-10-95 Ms. B saw the Dr. for the second time, at which time the Dr. prescribed 2 500 milligrams of M, per day, for 7 days. The Dr. took a genital culture during this visit. Since Ms. B had an obvious adverse reaction, a swollen face, to the original dosage of M, this writer advised her not to take this medication. Shortly thereafter, Ms. B was free of any vaginal problems. The Dr. had continued to attempt to prescribe M for Ms.B, at the wrong dosage, despite having received medical reports showing no vaginal bacteria problems. The Pap smear, taken on 02-22-95, found no endcervical cells. The report on the genital culture, taken on 03-10-95, reported that Ms. B had normal vaginal flora. One look at the dates and the continued attempts to use the drug M, on Ms. B, by this Dr., laid the foundation for possible serious cervical medical problems. M is well established as a treatment for protozoan infections, and for anaerobic bacterial infections. Per the drug mfg.. M was developed primarily for the treatment of T. Per the mfg,. the dosage for trichomonas vaginitis is 250 mg. of M, that should be taken by both the husband and the wife simultaneously for 10 days.

The drug manual lists vaginal inserts of 500mg. T causes a heavy discharge and is not rod shape. The normal bacteria, within the vagina, are of the bacillus type, which is a rod shape. The taking of M for a non-bacterial problem, at a higher than normal dosage, caused Ms. B to have a auto immune reaction that caused a swollen face and swollen bartholin B glands in the vagina. The swollen face was in reality swollen saliva glands. The swollen B glands blocked the normal lubricant from these glands that lubricate the vagina. As a result, the normal vagina bacteria balance was altered, along with a dry vagina, which lent itself to vaginal irritation. This leaves the bacillus bacteria in the vagina open to the adverse endospore/endotoxin process. This is the basis of a yeast infection as a result of the bacterial imbalance. The next media article that was significant was titled "CC is called fully preventable with routine use of pap smears, and safe sex the keys". Since the Dr. did not appear to want to report the adverse reaction, by Ms. B, to M, as required by the FDA, I went directly to the drug company. I received a letter from the drug company indicating that the package insert for M specifies that reactions may occur, such as urticaria (hives), and rashes. In the letter there was no mention of any swollen face reaction. I received a copy of the report to the FDA, by the drug company, and under the headings it indicated the use was for gardnerella vicinities, and the patient experienced a very swollen face, within 24 hours of ingestion, and the drug did not work for vaginal yeast infection. Also, it indicated under relevant history that the patient had no know allergies and yeast infection at the time of medication. Upon receiving this letter I contacted the sender and complained that the report never indicated the true problem, the misapplication and the wrong dosage of M. His response and or word's to the effect, "I don't care what the Doctors use it for and at what dosage"! He informed me that I was not to contact him anymore but to contact the legal dept. Similar to other contacts, during my fact-finding, when I received this type of response to my contact I immediately became suspicious of possible problems with M. I found a study in Scandinavia that says it all. In a study of 800 women, in Scandinavia, those women that took the drug M, for other than T, had high CC rates. I also found that if this or any other drug is misapplied, along with high dosages, it might cause serious medical problems. Finally, if the NH. Medical profession practices the same approach and treatment of a so called vaginal infection, such as experienced by Ms. B, by the Women Dr., in Nashua, I fully understand why NH. is first in CC cancer deaths and fourth in CC incidents in the nation.

Lung cancer in women

ABC's prime time nightly news had a piece on the epidemic in deaths among young women, from lung cancer. The piece indicated that there are more lung cancer deaths in young women (70,000) then the combine total from deaths from breast and ovarian cancers. Meanwhile, deaths from lung cancer, among men, have been steadily decreasing. They indicated that the medical establishment did not know the reason for these deaths. They mentioned that some of the symptoms were similar to asthma, (There has been a 62% increase in asthma over the last 10 years.) It stated that the medical people thought that pollutants may play a part in these deaths from lung cancer. I am sorry one doesn't have to go to medical school to realize that of course pollutants are involved. One look at the cancer deaths from smoking and passive smoke says it all.

Prior to providing details on the obvious inhaled pollution problems associated with these lung cancer deaths I believe the reader should become familiar with the body's respiratory process. Naturally, people are aware of the importance of oxygen, within the body's respiratory process, without realizing how complex the process is. The oxygen process is the union of a substance with oxygen that increases the positive valence and/or decreases the negative valence of an element or ion by the removal of electrons from atoms and or ions. For example: hydrogen or chlorine atoms making up H2O. Oxygen starvation may be based on genetics, where carboxyl hemoglobin is formed as a result of changes in the carbon to oxygen ration with an increase in C2O in the blood, thereby, reducing the free oxygen, thereby altering the depth and frequency of breathing, Oxygen starvation may be as a result of any one of the following: vasopressin's within food, drink, or drugs, toxins in the blood that interferes with the oxygen capacity of red blood cells, mucus within the wind pipe and or bronchial tube, particularly if toxic, may constrict blood vessels impeding the blood flow. Carboxyl hemoglobin is a compound that is formed in the blood when carbon monoxide, a highly poisonous gas, is created by the incomplete combustion of carbonaceous materials. The carbonaceous element occupies the position within the hemoglobin molecule normally taken by oxygen. The hydrolysis process carries oxygen from the lungs to the tissues and carbon dioxide away. Hemoglobin, acts to pick up oxygen where it is available and releases it where it is needed. Myoglobin on the other hand has a higher affinity for oxygen than does hemoglobin. Thus, even at relatively low partial pressures, myoglobin still tends to bind oxygen. In the respiratory system the air normally enters the respiratory system by way of the external nares or nostrils but it may also enter by way of the mouth. Molecules of oxygen and carbon dioxide diffuse readily through the thin, moist, walls of the alveoli. Each lung is covered by a thin sheet of smooth epithelium, the pleura. The pleura are kept moist, enabling the lungs to move without friction during breathing. Respiration also refers to the exchange of gases between the cells of an organism and the external environment. Many different methods for exchange are utilized by different organisms. Respiration may be categorized by three phases: external respiration, transportation by the bloodstream, and internal respiration. The process wherein the cells of an organism exchange oxygen and carbon dioxide directly, with the surrounding environment, is termed direct respiration. There are two types of neurons involved in the respiratory process. These two types of neurons are called insipiratory and expiratory neurons respectively. They also may be referred to as inspiratory and expiratory centers. When the inspiratory neurons are firing the expiratory center is prevented from firing so that expiration is inhibited. When inspiration ceases expiratory inhibition also stops. Respiration is stimulated by other factors aside from the variations in dissolved gas concentrations. Extremes of temperature, pain, initiation of exercise, and certain drugs, all act to stimulate respiration. Respiration, also changes with an individual's emotional state (possibly via hormonal changes), and may change by voluntary control.

The part that pollutants play in the death of young women, from lung cancer, may be evident in the data available. As previously indicated, lung cancer deaths from smoke says it all. Also, it is a fact that indoor pollution is 8x that of outdoor pollution. Also, as indicated, the symptoms at first are similar to asthma. Ironically, I believe the only reason for this reference to asthma was that the women, referenced, were all non smokers and didn't exhibit any smokers' symptoms. The symptoms described, for both these women and asthma, relate to the adverse reaction of the body's auto immune process as a result of the body ingesting a foreign agent and/or substance. In both cases, the adverse auto immune reaction causes an inflammation of the liquid glands of the body which in turn causes the reduction and/or the blockage of the associated liquids. This adverse reaction may cause a reduction in the breathing process from the swelling of the nasal passage, including the fossa. Also, the salivary glands may become swollen, shutting off all saliva, thereby creating a dry cough. In addition to the above, it was reported on, 03-21-04, that the carbon dioxide build up, in the, air has accelerated at a rapid rate. Since the body's adverse auto immune reaction is affected by the accumulation, compounding, and synergetic of all ingested agents and/or substances the carbon dioxide increase must be considered serious. This is particularly important when one recognizes the part C2O plays in the respiratory process itself. A good example is the airplane cold. Some people develop an airplane cold, with the dry cough, when they travel long distances in a large airplane. Airplane cold is caused by breathing in C2O from all the other passengers. This writer found that pollutants collected in my hair, along with pollutants transferred to the pillow case, caused adverse body reactions. I found the problem was compounded by the position I took, during the sleep cycle, particularly if my head was in a position to constantly inhale any pollutants in my hair and/or on the pillow case. Possibly, a woman would be more affected, during the sleep cycle, because they usually have more hair for the pollutant to collect in and in many cases they may have chemicals, including dyes, within their hair, and or on their bodies that may compound the problem. For an example of how the process works I would like to cite the example of this writer and a lady friend. I was traveling with a lady friend who I had not been with in several years. The first night we were preparing for bed, in our hotel room, I was standing directly behind her. She always wears a pony tail style, hair style, and she was releasing the pony tail in preparation for bed. I found that I had an adverse reaction to the pollutants, released from her hair. Ironically, it was not my imagination, that I had this adverse reaction. We had agreed, prior to the trip that she would only go on the trip with me if I did not talk about my findings on health care. So, when I had the adverse reaction to the pollutants in her hair I did not say a word but she said are you allergic to me? I still, as agreed upon, did not say one word. The pony tail style of hair is ideal for the collection of pollutants. Naturally, a person may be coming in contact with excessive amounts of CO, C2O, or chemicals, as a result of their work place and/or lifestyle. Finally, a look at a very important part of the overall process. As noted, each lung is kept moist, not only to enable it to function without friction, but to protect the lungs from any foreign agent and/or substance. Unfortunately, the body's adverse auto immune reaction could prevent the maintaining of the moist lung surfaces. Also, compounding the problem may be the drying effect the smoke vapors have on the lungs moist surfaces. In order for a woman to attempt to prevent lung cancer she must avoid all areas containing air pollution, particularly carbon monoxide. If for any reason she is unable to avoid any areas with high air pollution she must wash her hair and change her pillow case daily. This is particularly necessary among women who have a hair style that may capture pollutants such as a pony tail and/or a hair style of the hair down to the neck, style. Consider the alternatives; a woman may end up ingesting serious pollutants, all during the night, as she lay sleeping.

Colin

In the past when I was attempting to address a complicated medical problem I would always use the expression the possible cause and prevention of that medical problem. However, in regard to colon medical problems, I know definitely the cause and prevention of colon medical problems. Possibly, to attract the reader's interest in my findings they should consider two key factors. First, on a personal basis within about 12 hours from my last meal, I have no residue left within my colon that could breed any bacteria. Secondly, the would be residue that is eliminated, by at least two bowel movements, consists of a light colored, soft, non smelly stools (about ½ "wide and 12 "+ long). These bowel movements occur like clock work between 5 am, my wake up time, and 6:30 am … Most important, the process that this writer uses to assure the activation of these bowel movements is to activate the body's peristalsis process, that is associated with the body's autonomic process.

Diabetes

Per time magazine, "never have doctor's known so much about how to prevent or control this disease yet the epidemic keeps raging on". About 20.8 million Americans have one form or another of diabetes. About 6.2 million Americans don't know that they have diabetes. In 2002 there were 1.3 million new cases of diabetes, an increase of 878,000 from 1997. In 2002 about 200,000 Americans died from diabetes complications. The highest increases in incidents of diabetes are in developing nations, such as China. The medical scientific establishment (MSE) attempts to simplify the cause by stating that the epidemic of diabetes is caused by Americans eating too much and exercising too little. As a matter of fact Dr. Martin Silink, President, International Diabetes Foundation, is on record that diet is at fault. Unfortunately, it is more complicated than blaming those two factors. One look at the complicated process, involving the glucose in the blood, and it is easy to discount that diabetes is caused solely by over eating with too little exercise. The body regulates the amount of glucose in the blood like a fine tuned instrument. When the food is digested carbohydrates are split into glucose. This glucose is absorbed into the blood, where it is distributed to the liver and other organs. The liver automatically releases a certain amount of glucose into the blood, while at the same time saves a certain amount of glucose. At this point, the pancreas in its normal function releases insulin into the blood stream, with the amount regulated by the amount of glucose in the blood. The key is that the energy cells are activated by the insulin receptors which in turn allow the glucose to enter the cells. The (MSE) believe that this insulin/glucose process is governed by a genetic component and as a result a person may be predisposed to diabetes, as a result of the mother's metabolic and/or nutritional status during pregnancy. Type 1 diabetics have high glucose levels as a result of the inability of their pancreas to make insulin. Type 2 diabetics have faulty insulin receptors that prevent the opening of the cell. Also, the pancreas may not produce enough insulin. Regardless, glucose can't enter the cells and builds up in the blood. This writer believes that it is an adverse autoimmune reaction that directly affects the insulin/glucose process. As a matter of fact Time magazine, in its article on diabetes, listed seven conditions that may indicate that you have diabetes and five of the seven were adverse autoimmune reactions. The seven conditions were frequent urination, particularly at night, blurred vision, increased thirst, unusual hunger, unexplained weight loss, sores that do not heal and unusual fatigue. This writer believes that, even if you are genetically prone to diabetes, if you watch your diet, exercise, and do not ingest any agent and/or substance that may trigger your body's adverse auto immune reaction you may be able to avoid diabetes, particularly type 2. Finally, one must exercise to prevent diabetes.

Alzheimer's disease

A look at the unbelievable facts and figures related to Alzheimer's! Alzheimer's is a disease that may progress from a memory loss, to dementia, to death. At the present time, 4 million Americans are affected, with 3 million living at home. It causes about 100,000 deaths, and is the fourth leading cause of death. It affects about 10% of the population over 65, and 50% of the population over 85. It is expected that by the year 2028 there will be 16 million Americans affected by Alzheimer's disease. The key to properly addressing the Alzheimer's disease is the requirement to properly address the body's enzymes, as they relate to the metabolic digestive process. One look at some of the key factors, involving the body's enzymes, indicates how complicated this process is. High heats, such as 130o f, easily destroy enzymes! Natural foods have natural enzymes, and all cooked processed foods are devoid of their original enzymes. Also, the body's capacity to produce enzymes is limited. The body's metabolic digestive process starts within the mouth. It is the enzymes in the saliva, such as mucin, ptylin, and amylase that start the digestive/metabolic process! In regard to Alzheimer's the enzyme amylase is the key, since it hydrogenates the starch into maltose. The digestive enzyme secretions are regulated by neural factors, and by the molecules, in the ingested food, that stimulate receptor cells, to produce specific hormones, that circulate in the blood, until it reaches the secretors organs, which it controls. The control of secretions in digestion is a complex inter action of several factors, particularly, physical health, age, and diet. The process is completed when the pepsin enzyme, in the stomach, splits the long protein into shorter fragments or peptides that are further digested in the intestines! The acidity of the stomach inhibits the action of the amylase enzyme, leaving most of the starch undigested. It is not until the starch reaches the small intestines, that another amylase, secreted by the pancreas, finishes the metabolism, of starch into maltose.

At this point, it should be obvious to the reader, that if for any reason a problem develops, within the body, involving amounts and timeliness, of key enzymes, the body's metabolic digestive process may be adversely affected!. One such problem is called the body's auto immune system! The body's auto immune process acts adversely to what it perceives as an ingested pollutant, to the accumulation, compounding, and or synergetic of a particular agent and/or substances, within the air, food, drink, and/or medications. This adverse auto immune reaction causes the swelling of one or more of the body's liquid glands! As a result, the fluids from these glands, that include key enzymes, such as the amylase, are either reduced in flow and/or the flow is blocked completely. When this happens to the amylase it not only interferes with the digestive process but in turn fails to hydrogenate the starch into sugar. As a result, a condition develops called amyloidosis, which in reality is unmetabolized starch that becomes a plaque! Also, while this process is taking place it is possible that the body will attempt to make a normal correction that may result in beta amyloidal, 1 which is a super plaque. This plaque clogs the arteries in the brain, and causes a lack of oxygen, which is the precursor to Alzheimer's.

Recently, a study was conducted among about 90 men and women with the average age 67, titled "Failure to identify odors linked to Alzheimer's", on the possible correlation between a loss of smell and the onset of Alzheimer's! The study found that many of the people, in the study, reported no problems with smell, prior to the study, but were found to have smell problems in the study. Also, a large segment of these people developed Alzheimer's disease. Normally, I am rather skeptical about many studies conducted by the medical establishment in support of this or that theory, however; in this case I am able to personally confirm their findings. A few years ago I was diagnosed with the rare disorder called Sjogren Syndrome. The medical establishment suspected that it was associated with the body's immune system, but did not know what caused it! I found that the cause of my Sjogren Syndrome was an adverse reaction to excessive amounts of whey in margarine! I developed severely swollen saliva glands. In retrospect it, was obvious that I had years of adverse autoimmune problems. In particular, I had problems with my smell, as a result of the damage to my olfactory nerve from repeated inflammations. I also experienced short-term memory problems. In my opinion if the doctor, in the emergency room, had not discovered the cause of my swollen saliva glands, Sjogren Syndrome, I would be directly affected by the Alzheimer's disease today. Summing up my findings, if any person experiences an ongoing dry throat, and/or swollen saliva glands, that person has ingested a pollutant that has caused an auto immune reaction that blocked the amylase which in turn results in unmetabolized starch that turns into a super plaque! This plaque clogs the arteries causing oxygen starvation to the brain hence Alzheimer's.

Connective tissue disease

While there are several diseases associated with what is referred to as connective tissue disease the one type of connective tissue disease that stands out is arthritis. I believe that the article in the media, written by a doctor, explained the process accurately. The article indicated that the connective tissue is formed by collagen, a fibrous protein, which is also found in large quantities in ligaments, cartilage, muscles, and bone. It went on to say that when inflammation strikes at this tissue it's known as connective tissue disease. It further stated that the cause of the inflammation is not completely understood, but it may be associated with an autoimmune response. What was not addressed was the fact that while the tissue itself is inflamed, the synovial fluid, in the joints, is reduced and or blocked entirely, thereby contributing to the restricted movement of the joint. There are three different types of joints where arthritis strikes. Arthritis is defined as pain, inflammation and stillness in one or more joints. Joints are the connections between two bones. By allowing one bone to move in relation to the bone next to it, joints permit a wide range of motion. The different bones of a joint are held together by connective tissue strands called ligaments. Skeletal muscles, attached to the bones by means of another type of connective tissue strand known as a tendon, produce their effects by bending the skeleton at the movable joints. The ends of each bone at a movable joint are covered with a layer of smooth cartilage. These bearing surfaces are completely enclosed in a liquid-tight capsule, called the bursa. The joint cavity is filled with a liquid lubricant, called, the synovial fluid, which is secreted by the membrane lining. During youth and early maturity the lubricant is replaced as needed, but in middle and old age the supply is often decreased, resulting in joint stiffness and difficulty of movement. A common disability known as bursitis is due to the inflammation of cells lining the bursa, and also results in restrained movement. The vertebrates are characterized by having an endoskeleton—a bony or cartilaginous framework lying within the body—surrounded by muscles. The arthropods, on the other hand, have an exoskeleton. The arthropod exoskeleton is a chitinous framework on the outside of the body surrounding the muscles. The contraction of muscles in the verte-brates moves one bone with respect to another. One end of the muscle is attached to one bone and the other end is attached to another bone. While there is some thought process among the (MSE) that arthritis may be genetically connected this writer, based on my own personal experience, has to attribute arthritis to the body's adverse autoimmune reaction. Every one of my family members, mother and father, and seven siblings, has contracted arthritis, while this writer has not contracted arthritis. Also, I believe that, at times, when I eat something that I shouldn't, particularly in large quantities I believe I feel arthritic type symptoms in my right knee.

Heart disease

While there are several various types of heart diseases this writer will only attempt to address only two, coronary artery disease, and atrial fibrillation. (Irregular heart beat and/or abnormal cardiac rhythm). It is important to note that while we usually relate to a heart attack when referencing heart disease there are 450,000 deaths, per year, from irregular heart beats. A few factors to consider, in the addressing the cause of heart disease, are that high blood pressure affects 9 out of 10 middle age Americans. Also, in a recent study by the AMA of 230 patients, overall, 37% had heart muscles damaged by exposure to carbon monoxide. The heart damaged often caused no initial symptoms, but was detected by hospital tests. Also, it was reported that the immune system may play a role in heart dis-ease. In the report it indicated that macrophages, large wandering cells, capable of engulfing and devouring bacteria and other foreign invaders, within the body's immune system, may be capable of developing certain forms of heart disease. The process involves atherosclerotic plaque. The atherosclerotic plaque is the fatty material deposited on the interior surface of an artery. As it builds up it clogs the artery, reducing the blood transporting ability of the vessel, and paving the way for a heart attack. As noted, plaque may break away and cause a blood clot. As noted, clogging and high blood pressure goes hand in hand. In coronary artery disease, this writer believes that the number one cause is clogged arteries. The clogged arteries may be traced back to diet, in association with the body's adverse auto immune process. Atrial fibrillation is a condition: of rapid, uneven, contrac-tions, within the upper heart chambers (atria). This causes the lower heart cham-ber (ventricles) to beat irregularly, at the rate of 130 to 150 per minute. The lower chamber cannot contract in response to all these impulses, and the contractions become disordered. The upper chamber may discharge more than 350 electric impulses per minute. The rapid pulsations results in decreased amounts of blood pumped to the body. This may cause blood clots to form in the upper heart chamber. The most common causes of atrial fibrillation are, high blood pressure, coronary artery disease, chronic lung disease, and pulmonary embolism.. This writer found that be it coronary and/or atrial heart problems they are related to the clogging of the arteries which in turn are related to a person's diet including excessive quantities of caffeine, alcohol, and so called inactive agents within food, drink, and medications. The reader should be aware that the most dangerous drug on the market is the blood thinning drug. Only take this drug as a last resort, and only after having it prescribed by two different doctors.

Asthma

In a 2004 report it was reported that 16 million adults and 9 million children were suffering from respiratory illnesses and/or asthma. It was estimated that the health costs, associated with asthma, was costing American's 1.3 billion. Per the medical scientific establishment (MSE) there are three mysteries involving asthma. First, is its root cause, second, how to treat it, thirdly, why has the number of asthma sufferers increased so quickly? The MSE is quoted as saying that 20 to 30 years ago asthma was a disease one saw only occasionally. In one article, on the possible causes of asthma, it listed dust mites, mold, pets, pollen, roaches, and smoke. Once again in that article, it was all about allergic reactions, associated with asthma, and nothing about the body's adverse autoimmune process. This writer found that, in some people, there is an inflammation of the respiratory tract from an autoimmune reaction to something they have ingested from the air, food, drink and/or from the so called inactive agents in medications. However, the primary source of the cause of asthma is the mold/fungus vapor ingested by a person, within old buildings and/or slums, and/or buildings located in predominately hot humid climates. One look at the states with the highest asthma rates, all in New England, ties in with the older buildings and asthma. Also, it was found that the asthma rates were higher in the slums of most large cities. This writer believes that the slum dwellers suffer from asthma because of the mold/fungus, and filth present in the older homes of slum dwellers that are in homes locked up tight, for security purposes, without adequate air. I also believe that another reason for the severe changes in the asthma rate from 20 years ago is the fact that people spend more time indoors, particularly in these mold infested homes, because of TV's, and changes in life styles. Also, once again there are medications, on the market, that may react in conjunction with the mold/fungus, thereby, causing asthma. In one case it was found that the use of melatonin, to induce sleep, kept asthmatics up all night. The only solution to solving the asthma problem is called clean up and/or clean out the mold/fungus. For an example of how this may work I cite the example of the thrift shop, at the senior center. A few people who began their bridge game in the room adjoining the thrift shop, which was closed between 12 noon and 1 0" clock, had an asthmatic type reaction when the door to the thrift shop opened at 1 o'clock. This reaction was caused by the mold vapor off of the donated clothing. Once the windows of the thrift shop were opened, to air out the thrift shop the smell went away. Naturally, some people might be exposed to the mold/fungus conditions in schools, churches, and in the home. Also, it is necessary to use bleach in all drains and areas where mold/fungus may collect. Along with these steps, I believe, based on this writer's personal experience, one has to change the pillow case frequently, since pollution may be transferred from the hair to the pillow case.. Also, this writer found that mold/fungus collects within stuff chairs.

Yeast infections

This writer concurred with the medical profession that yeast infections are caused by the disturbance of the bacterial balance process, within the vagina. The bartholin's glands are the key. These glands consist of two small glands on each side of the base of the vagina. Its function is to secrete mucus that assists in maintaining the bacterial balance in the vagina. If this bacterial (bacillus) balance is disturbed, by any metallic type agents, including from medications, it will allow the yeast to grow and take over the vagina. To prevent yeast infections, one must not introduce any metallic type materials into the vagina. A good example of how the process works is to look at the requirements to maintain the bacterial balance within a successful septic tank. Anyone familiar with the process realizes that one should not allow colored toilet paper to enter the septic tank process since it will alter the bacterial balance causing the septic tank process to malfunction.

Autism

This writer feels that there are at least two causes of autism. The number one cause is the pregnant women inhaling excessive amounts of carbon monoxide during pregnancy. There has been a 270% increase in autism in California with only one conclusion for this dramatic increase, air pollution. Also, it was reported that an EPA office in a large eastern city found excessive amounts of birth defects among its employees. This writer believes the cause was the enclosed, with no vents, underground garage, with two large elevators that opened at the garage level, allowing the excessive carbon monoxide to go right up the elevator into the work areas. The other cause of autism is the metals in the vaccines given to children. In particular, it was found that thimerosal, a mercury-based preservative, in children's vaccines, may be responsible for the increase in autism, attention deficit disorders, and other childhood neurological disorders, among children. The above conditions can only be prevented by the elimination of the agents involved, not by the use of any medications. In the case of the problems with the reaction to metals in the vaccines it is associated with the endospore/endotoxin process.

Airplane cold

Within the human body's respiratory process a carbon dioxide CO_2 (a colorless gas with a anthracite base) is expired. During any long airplane trip problems may develop among some passengers with so many people expiring CO_2 in an enclosed space. When most people ingest this CO_2 they develop a so-called airplane cold. To immediately correct this airplane cold all one has to do is, upon leaving the plane, and in a relatively open space, inhale and exhale large amounts of air. This will return the person to a normal breathing cycle.

Loss of taste or smell

In taste, the ingested agents and/or substances contact the tongue and send nerve impulses to a special taste center in the cortex (outer layer of the brain), and the thalamus (a pair of large oval organs forming part of the brain). These organs are made up of grey substances that translate impulses, from the receptors for pain, temperature, and touch. It also involves mechanisms that produce reflex movements of the brain. The key enzyme in the saliva and in the taste buds is the ptyalin, that primarily aides in the breakdown of starch. The front of the tongue is most sensitive to sweets and salty substances. The sides of the tongue are most sensitive to bitter substances. The middle of the tongue produces no taste. In smell, there is a smell sensing area in the chamber behind the nose (nasal cavity), that contains the olfactory nerve (one of a pair of nerves linked to the sense of smell). It is made up of many thin threads that spread through the mucus membrane, of the smell sensing areas in the nasal cavity, and passes into the skull. The fibers form links, with the fibers, of the cells, in the olfactory bulb. This is a relay center for the cranial nerve, or a relay between the nose and the brain part, responsible for being aware of odors. This writer found that certain adverse autoimmune reactions caused the inflammation of the taste buds and/or the more complicated olfactory nerve, which in turn are damaged and/or destroyed, thereby, directly affecting one's sense of smell and/or taste. Compounding the above problem takes place when the same adverse autoimmune reaction inflames the saliva glands, thereby, blocking and/or destroying enzymes involving the smell and taste process. While the causes of the loss of taste and/or smell are very similar, the causes of the loss of smell are more involved and detailed. Anoosimiag, a loss and/or damage of the sense of smell is usually temporary, but may become permanent when any part of the olfactory nerve is destroyed by long term inflammation.

Sjogren syndrome (SS)

The real turning point in this writer's fact finding came when this writer was diagnosed with a rare disorder called SS. Up to this point, since I had no know medical problems, in fact I did not require an aspirin, it was hard to relate to my various contact's medical problems! It was almost as if I purposely planned to have a problem with SS in order to relate to others! Most important, I became familiar with the body's autoimmune process! Prior to being diagnosed with SS, and its tie in with the body's autoimmune process, I was confused as to what I thought was an allergic reaction! The reaction, while appearing to be an allergic reaction, did not involve the usual histamine flow! Also, in retrospect, I found that over the years I developed reactions to agents that previously I had no reaction too! My confusion was resolved when in June of 1999 I went to an allergy Doctor with a swollen face thinking it was some sort of allergy! The Doctor informed me that it was not an allergy, but offered no other advice as to the possible cause! I next went to my personal care physician PCP, who also did not know the cause of my swollen face, but offered to medicate me! I then went to an emergency room ER at an out of state hospital, since my PCP was not about to direct me to a specialist! A women doctor, in the ER, felt that I had a rare disorder and sent me to a specialist within the hospital. The specialist indicated to me that the swollen face was really swollen saliva glands which were one of the symptoms of SS! A review of the various body reactions to SS and it was obvious that not only had I been experiencing problems with SS but it accounted for my apparent so-called allergic reactions! I also identified several symptoms that were not listed as related to SS! The biggest shocker was that the MSE&AF did not know what caused SS; they thought it was associated with the body's immune system! They did not know how to treat it! I traced my problem with SS to the excessive use of margarine, in particular the whey in the margarine! I had an auto immune reaction to the whey! Finally, I was able to differentiate between an allergic reaction and an auto immune reaction and I was able to correct the problem by the elimination of the agent and/or substance within my food, drink, and/or in the air, that caused the body's adverse auto immune reaction, resulting in SS. A summary of the types of the body's adverse reaction to SS are as follows: vertigo, dry eyes, dry mouth and dry skin, along with a swollen bladder that reduces the capacity of the bladder. In women, they may experience a dry vagina, which is caused by the swollen bartholin glands that in turn reduces and/or blocks the lubricant and thereby causing irritation and infection. The dry skin is a precursor to the scleroderma disease.

Special note nine times more women than men develop this disorder

Scleroderma

This is a disease that affects the body's blood vessels and connective tissue. It features a fibrous breakdown of tissue in the skin, lungs, and other internal organs. It occurs more often in middle age women. This disease is associated with Sjogren Syndrome. By preventing Sjogren Syndrome, as outlined in the article on the cause and prevention of Sjogren Syndrome, one will automatically prevent scleroderma.

World wide obesity

Background In a report published by the Associated Press, it indicated that an obesity pandemic threatens to overwhelm health systems around the world. The World Health Organization says more than 1 billion adults are overweight, and 300 million of them are obese, putting them at a much higher risk of diabetes, heart problems, high blood pressure, strokes and some forms of cancer. Not only is obesity prevalent among the overeating wealthy people, but it is prevalent among some of the poorest people. For example, Thailand's Public Health Ministry announced that nearly one in three Thais, over age 35, is at risk, of obesity related diseases. In the report, it indicated that one of the most worrying problems are the skyrocketing rates of obesity, among children, which makes them much more prone to chronic diseases as they grow older and could shave years off their lives, experts said. The national obesity rate is 32%. Obesity rates climbed in 31 states with the Colorado rate 17.6% and the district of Columbiathe highest percentage with 22.8% among children ages 10 to 17.

Process First of all a body mass index greater than 30 is considered to be obese. This index is a ratio height and weight. Obesity results from the limited ability of the body to store proteins and carbohydrates therefore excess food in any form is coverted into stored fat. This problem is compounded if the person in question has a genetic metabolism abnormally. Naturally, while this person is ingesting excessive food and not burning any calories it means obesity.

Preventing obesity Normally, when I am acquiring documented data in support of a particular medical finding in most cases I have to go to more than one source. In regard to the World wide obesity problem I only had to go to a single source, Japan. Japan is not only the healthiest nation in the world, but it has no obesity. Recognizing that Japan was the healthiest nation in the world I visited with them to find out why. I found out that there were two major factors were involved in their becoming the healthiest nation in the world. Ironically in turn these two factors also prevented obesity in Japan.

The first factor is **DIET**. The Japanese diet consists of very little red meat, but if eaten, it is always eaten without starch.(attached Pancreas) It is composed of skinless raw fruits and vegetables, particularly leafy vegetable s on a daily basis. The Japanese food is always warm never hot (not over 130 degrees) so that none of the enzymes and/or vitamins are lost from over heating. The diet allows for the enzymes and the vitamins, in the raw food, to digest very efficiently, within the stomach, so that the calories are burned efficiently. One of the key enzymes is called celluse, an inert carbohydrate. This enzyme breaks down the fibers of whole grains, vegetables, fruits, and nuts that normally resist digestion in the gastrointestinal tract. As a result, a person doesn't experience the gastric ills of putrefaction (an action that causes matter to rot and/or decompose, particularly proteins and organic matter, with the production of foul smelling compounds such as hydrogen sulfate, ammonia, and mercaptans), and fermentation, as in yeast enzymes, molds, and certain bacteria,(an action that decomposes carbohydrates that in turn form acetic, butyric, and/or lactic acids). The Japanese feel strongly that their ingesting of ample amounts of fiber has contributed to their good health. The fibers involved consist of carbohydrates, such as celluse or pectin and in particular amorphous colloidal carbohydrate that occur in fruits especially apples.

The second factor is **LIFESTYLE**. Unlike the Chinese the Japanese have no fast food establishments. This eliminates fried foods with its trans fat. They daily assist in the body's peristalsis process thereby providing excellent waste elimination. They have very few autos on the road, using public transportation with its walking exercise. and lack of air pollution..

Skin eruptions

The skin consists of many layers of cells. The thin outer layer, epidermis, which is free of blood vessels, and the dermis, an inner thick layer, which is packed with blood vessels and nerve endings, The epidermis outer layer is stratified epithelium whose thickness varies in different parts of the body. It is thickest on the soles of the feet, palms of the hands, and contains dead skin with large amounts of fibrous protein. This protein regulates heat loss and sweating, which excretes 5 to 10 % of all metabolic waste. Sweat is the same as urine, but it is much more diluted. Within the skin are melanocytes cells that produce the pigment melanin, that absorbs ultraviolet rays. Keratin is a scieroprotein or albuminoid substance found in the dead outer skin layer, and in horns, hair, feathers, hoofs, nails, claws, bills, etc., Albiminoid, also called scleroprotien, is any of a class of simple proteins, such as keratin, gelatin, or collagen, that are insoluble in all neutral solvents. Melanin is a pigment excreted by the melanocyte cells and is any of a class of insoluble pigments found in all forms of animal life that account for the dark color of skin, hair, fur, scales, feathers, etc.. Mucin, is any of a class of glycoprotiens found in salvia). gastric juices, etc., that form viscous solutions and acts as a lubricant or protectant, on external and internal surfaces of the body. (Also found in the main part of mucus where it protects the skin from abrasions) Glycoprotein, is a group of complex proteins, such as mucin, containing a carbohydrate, combined with a simple protein. Skin eruptions are caused by the blocking and or the reduction of key skin chemicals such as mucin and keratin. Also, a genetic problem may be involved with the improper production of melanin resulting in skin eruptions. Finally, in some people excessive exposure to ultraviolet rays especially over a long period may not just cause skin eruptions but cause skin cancer.

SKIN PROBLEMS: The blocking of the mucin, and/or melanin, may result in skin cancer. Keratitis is the inflammation of the cornea of the eye as a result of the body's adverse autoimmune reaction. Many years of over exposure to sunlight may cause precancerous keratonic lesions.(commonly called senile keratoses) British skin results in skin cancer deaths in Great Britain In some people, with British skin, the melanin is not uniform throughout a particular layer of the skin, such as the face, thereby exposing the skin to the ultraviolet rays. Finally, there is the rare disorder Scleroderma, a skin disease, associated with the body's adverse autoimmune process and prevented by eliminating ingesting certain agents and/ or substances.

Aging

It has been found that older people have more diabetes than younger people. Study's found that the inability of older people to process sugar, optimally, was caused not by age alone. The study found that, as one grows older, there is a loss of lean bodyweight, sometimes as much as 30%. That the loss of lean body weight, and the corresponding increase in body fat, along with the redistribution of the body fat, coupled at times with physical inactivity, causes some of the body's systems to go out of balance. As a result, there are fewer cells left in the body for burning energy. The circulatory system has a reduced ability to carry drugs (genitourinary sites for elimination)! The metabolic rate decreases, causing the blood flow to decrease. Also, because of the higher ratio of fat cells, in an older person's body, many drugs that are soluble in fat might linger longer and cause adverse body reactions. If the drug lingers too long, any ingestion of multiple drugs may cause an adverse reaction with each other. Oxygen to the blood is slower in the aged. Any decrease in the metabolism rate means a decrease in the blood flow. Movement into the stomach takes more time, since peristalsis contractions lessen,* because of the loss of tone and a reduction in the stimulation of the nervous system. A decrease in gastric gland secretions causes a decrease in the absorption of some nutrients and medications. Age slows down the flow of microbobialflo, which assists in digestion and metabolism. Too little fat, 20% or less of calories, may cause the metabolic rate to become distorted with trans fat, a toxic substance, becoming a fact, causing the liver to produce more rather than less bad cholesterol! Despite all the possible adverse body reactions, indicated in the above, I believe it is possible for a person to compensate for these aging processes. First, if a person is born with the proper basic enzymes this may slow the aging process. Secondly, if a person practices proper dietary habits, including excluding ingesting any agents that might trigger the body's adverse auto immune reaction, where the key enzymes are blocked and/or reduced in flow, I believe the aging process will be lessened. In particular, there are three enzymes directly related to the condition of the body's face, which is usually the main indicator of aging. Those enzymes are melanin, which absorbs the ultra violet rays, mucin, that lubricates the skin and keratin, a protein that provides body to the skin without causing any puffiness of the skin. Added to these processes is the exercise process that not only helps to maintain the body's overall muscle tone, but assists in the proper internal chemical reactions from the body's digestive process, to the body's elimination process. However, despite anyone adhering to all of the above suggestions it still helps if a person inherits their Mother's British skin! Unfortunately, it was found that in the British skin the melanin is not evenly distributed through out the skin thereby leaving openings where the ultra violet light may penetrate causing skin cancer!

Steps to prevent aging Avoid ingesting pollutants within the air, foods, drinks, and drugs. Implement the Japanese diet. Exercise, by at least walking, five times per week. Daily conduct deep breathing exercises

The sleep cycle

60% of all Americans claim that they have an improper sleep cycle! It has been reported that 30 million Americans, more than 1 in 10, suffer specifically from chronic insomnia. Studies in the 1990s estimated that the cost of medical care for sleep disorders is $15.9 billion. Naturally, the foremost cause of an adverse sleep cycle might be a medical problem, affecting one or more physical parts of the body, including the brain. Possibly, the next prominent factors adversely affecting the sleep cycle are the body's improper digestion and/or metabolism along with the body's improper waste elimination! As a result of the failure of these processes pressure is put on the bowels, and the bladder, that affects the sleep cycle! The problems are compounded, at night, since the associated muscles are relaxed! Also, any attempt to address these factors with medications, in many cases only makes the problem worse, since the medications may cause an auto immune reaction! (The problem is also compounded if a person wears tight night clothing around the body's midsection). Finally, even if the above factors are properly addressed there is still the body's melatoning process that needs to be properly addressed. Melatonin (a hormone) secreted by the pineal gland into the blood or lymph) in an inverse proportion to the amount of light received by the retina upon the onset of darkness. This signals the body of the appearance of a sleep factor. Also, it initiates the body's biorhythm process (an innate periodicity physical process in the body's sleep/awake cycle), where a particular body forms its own innate periodicity as to the sleep/awake cycle. Similar to other body processes the process itself may be adversely affected by any melatonin supplements. It was reported that in one case a small amount of a melatonin supplement caused the inflammation of the airways! This is a autoimmune reaction to the total amount of melatonin, from the body itself, along with the supplement! Since, the body normally increases melatonin production, with the onset of darkness, signaling the approach of sleep, international travel, particularly traveling east, plays havoc with the normal sleep/awake cycle. It was found that after a long eastbound trip the melatonin virtually stops for days resulting in what some people call jet lag! This writer's sleep/awake cycle is as a result of having established, via the body's innate biorhythm process, a periodicity physical process. This process, in conjunction with the body's autonomic process, provided this writer with a definitive sleep/awake cycle. Don't place the bed covers above the neck in order to prevent the possible containment of the breath's expiration of carbon dioxide that could be inhaled! Also, one must wear warm night clothing, particularly on the body's upper parts. This is necessary because of the body's normal movement, during the sleep cycle, causing the blankets to be disturbed thereby exposing the body to possible cold air! A normal sleep cycle may be assisted by the body's position while sleeping. If possible sleep on your side, flexing your knees so that they are almost even with your stomach. This position is similar to the body's sitting position that restricts the urinary muscles while sitting. Use a pillow and/or pillows that allows for a slight up angle of the head. This allows for proper breathing during the sleep cycle. In addition to the above, the media recently reported that a leading actress just had a nose job. The actress reported that she did not have a nose job on the nose itself, but had her deviated septum taken care of. She said that she now sleeps much better at night.

Finally practice the mediation process while in bed just prior to going to sleep.

Over active bladder

One out of every three women over forty five suffer from urinary incontinence. 1.9 billion Adult diapers were sold in 2002. In 1961 only 10% of all two and one-half year olds were still in diapers. By the year 1997 78% of all two and one-half year olds were still in diapers. First of all, when one reads that a person has urinary problems as a result of an over active bladder this is not totally correct. Any release of urine from the bladder is controlled by the body's autonomic process (see definition in chapter on body processes), and the capacity of the bladder to hold urine. Compounding the above is the fact that, at night, the controlling muscles, involving the urinary tract, assumes a relaxed mode, with very little and/ or no individual body control. If a person has no infection, along the urinary tract and/or prostate problems, and that person has a urinary problem it is normally as a result of several possible causes. First, there is the under capacity of the bladder as a result of the inflammation of the bladder. The main reason for the under capacity of the bladder is that the bladder is affected by an adverse autoimmune reaction (see definition in chapter on body processes) causing the bladder to swell up, thereby, reducing the bladder's capacity to hold urine. As far back as the 1920's and1930's doctors found that certain children lost urinary control and wet the bed when they ate certain foods, but had perfect control when they avoided these foods. This writer was a late bed wetter, as a child, and to this day I find that if I eat certain foods I have to get up more than once, during the night, to rush to urinate. Naturally, this is the body's adverse autoimmune process that may be triggered by, not only certain foods, but by other ingested agents and/or substances. This writer found that I had an autoimmune reaction to cat dander (protein in cat saliva), on my bed clothing, that forced me to get up several times, during the night, to urinate. In conjunction with the above factors, affecting urinary incontinence, this writer found that if I had pressure from tight clothing across the urinary tract, and/or did not dress warm across the urinary tract, I would have problems with urinary incontinence. This process was compounded when the same adverse autoimmune process, indicated in the above, caused a swollen sphincter muscle and/or the urethra, thereby causing an interruption in the urinary flow. My personal experience illustrates how the above process works. I had a salad, with nothing but regular vegetables and natural mayonnaise. I also had pickle slices from a jar of pickles. Immediately, I had to run to the bathroom to urinate. It was obvious that I had a reduced capacity bladder, from a swollen bladder, caused by an adverse auto immune reaction.(AAR). At first, I could not understand what was causing my problem until I read the information on the pickle jar. I called the product manager, of a well known pickle company, and asked him why he had the strongest preservative on the market, titanium dioxide, in the pickle jar, that contained vinegar, and that had to be refrigerated after opening? His response was, "to maintain the color of the pickles." Possibly, two of the most significant causes of urinary incontinence are as follows: A person can't allow a build up along the alimentary canal of solid waste since the pressure on the urinary tract could cause urinary problems. At the present time this writer eats a lot of fiber in my diet and I attempt prior to bed time to eliminate any intestinal gas. I eat my main meal at noon time, which consists of chicken and/or turkey and/or non red meat. At the same time, I have a salad of raw vegetables. In the late afternoon, I eat at least one apple, depending on the size of the apples. As a result of the above, after going to sleep about 9:30 pm I awake at about 12pm to urinate as a result of the relaxing of the muscles from the body's autonomic process. Upon returning to bed I immediately fall back to sleep. I awake about 5:00 am to urinate and to have breakfast. I have a normal bowel movement, like clockwork, sometime between 5:00 am and 6:00 am. I usually have a second bowel movement shortly after my lunch. Finally, one should pay attention to the body's autonomic process at night, relative to urinary incontinence. First of all, a person doesn't have control, day or night, over the body's autonomic process, which controls the body's urinary process. However, the problem is compounded at night, since during the sleep process the urinary tract muscles are relaxed. Therefore, a person should expect to, at times, get up at night to urinate. However, this event usually occurs more frequently in an older a person as a result of the aging muscles, and their reaction to the cold. So, if you take drugs for a so called over active bladder, when it is the normal aging problem, you may prevent getting up more frequently to urinate, but you might develop medical problems from the medication. If I lay on my back, during the night, it is almost as if I am telling my body, urinate all night. I believe one should lie on their side with the knees flexed up so that they are almost even with the stomach. This position is similar to the body's sitting position that restricts the urinary muscles.

Liver

Liver is the body's metabolic headquarters. It is directly responsible for a person's overall sense of well being and vitality. During periods of rest, especially in cold weather, 30% to 50% of the body's blood supply collects in the liver and pancreas. During the sleep cycle, the blood is fortified, in the liver, for the use by the rest of the body. During activity, when a person moves blood moves, and when a person is still the blood returns to the liver. The liver is the site of the synthesis of a host of blood proteins, and where cholesterol is made. For blood, protein, fat, and sugar, it plays a role analogous to that of the kidney, for Ions. Also, it acts not only for circulatory connections, but for digestive-gallbladder and intestines connections. Bile, which it exports, contains a substance that acts as a detergent to help break up the fat globules, in the intestines. The major bile pigment is bilirubin, a breakdown product of hemoglobin, the oxygen carrying protein red blood cells. The liver constantly secretes bile (600-800 ml. per day). A network of ducts collects the bile and passes it into the gallbladder where it is stored until needed. When food enters the duodenum certain receptor cells, in the duodenum, secrete a hormone called cholecystokinin (CCK) into the blood stream. In the wall, of the intestine, it senses the presence of fats in the chime that in itself is stimulated by fats. Chime is the thick gummy contents of the stomach during the digestion of food. This hormone causes the inhibition of gastric motility and contractions of the gallbladder, forcing bile out through the bile duct and into the small intestine. If, the bile duct is blocked, so that pigments can't be excreted in the bile, they will be reabsorbed into the liver causing liver problems. Bile is very important for proper digestion, although it contains no enzymes! It is highly alkaline, and helps neutralize the acid, in the chime, as it leaves the stomach and enters the small intestines. This is necessary in order for the intestinal enzymes to function. Bile is composed of bile salt, lecithin, cholesterol, and bile pigment. The first three are involved in the emulsification of fat, in the small intestine. The bile pigment gives bile its color. Bile salts are the most active part of bile. These salts are essential for the digestion of fats. Butter & oil are fats, which constitute part of a group of molecules called lipids. Lipids are insoluble in water and tend to coalesce to form globules. The enzyme, that digests lipids, called lipases, can only work on the surface of these globules. Alone it would take weeks for lipases to complete fat digestion in this manner. Bile salts solve this problem by acting as a detergent, breaking the globules into million of tiny droplets, called micelles. This process called emulsification greatly increases the surface area exposed to attack, by the lipases, speeding up lipid digestion. Bile salts are conserved by the body and are reabsorbed in the lower part of the intestines, and carried back to the liver, through the blood stream, and secreted again. The liver excretes excess cholesterol in the bile. The prevention of liver problems is the proper function of the bile process. Also, avoid eating too much wheat (gluten) since it may adversely affect the function of the liver.

Sinus

When this writer was a young man I had sinus trouble so bad that the pressure within my sinus cavity dictated the comings and goings of all the changes in the weather. The degree of pressure, within my sinus cavity, was directly related to the changes in the atmosphere with respect to wind, temperature, cloudiness, moisture, and particularly air pressure. If the weather person appeared to hesitate as to the extent of the degree of changes in the weather I would know the degree of change by the effect on my sinus cavity. I also experienced breathing problems, similar to asthma, from the mucus within the respiratory passages. During my youth, particularly while I was very active in sports that included football, hockey, and baseball, it was natural for me to become distracted by my severe sinus condition. At that time I had many opportunities to talk with members of the medical profession about my sinus condition. All my contacts would respond with the comment that they did not know what to do about my sinus condition. In some cases the medical contact had sinus problems themselves. Once out in the business world I not only continued to experience my sinus problems, but at times my problems became worse because of other pollutants in the air. Despite my previous lack of help, from the medical profession, on solving my sinus problems, I decided to try one more time to seek help. I went to a doctor and explained my problems with my sinus cavity. He took one look up my nostrils and declared that we will try to help you by taking care of that deviated septum. The septum is the hard tissue that separates the two nostrils. Some people are born with a deviated septum, while others may have injured the septum, so that it is curved, blocking one of the nostrils. During an office visit, the Doctor went into the nostril and with a scalpel cut out the deviated septum that was blocking the nostril. The results were immediate, no more sinus and/or breathing problems period.

Sciatic nerve

The sciatic nerves are a pair of nerves that are the largest in the body and that originate in the sacral plexus of the lower back, and extend down the buttocks to the back of the knees. Any pain or tenderness from these nerves is usually caused by a prolapsed (a falling down of the vertebra (bones of the spinal column) affecting the intervertebral disk (the plate of fibrocartilage between the vertebra). While to the best of my knowledge despite many years of sports I did not seem to be bothered by sciatic nerve problems. However, after several years removed from my sports days I ran into a sciatic nerve problems. I had a very important sales meeting that I had to attend, but I had very severe sciatic nerve problem. I was living in Chicago, at the time, and had to fly out of O'Hare field to the sales meeting. The pain was so bad that I had my wife drive me to the airport, while I was on my knees, facing backwards, in the passenger seat. When I returned home, from the sales meeting, I immediately went to a Doctor. I explained to the Doctor my problems with my severe back pain and asked him if he could help me. He casually said well we could try this and see if it helps. He told me to get up and lay on my back on the table. He told me to rise up and touch my toes. I did what he told me without any pain. Subsequent to that time I have performed that exercise on a daily basis and have never had any more sciatic nerve pain period. It was obvious that this exercise opened up the vertebra, which took pressure off the disk that in turn prevented the disk from putting pressure on the sciatic nerve. When I went to my 50th high school class reunion so many people, many who I barely knew while in school, commented on how they thought I got taller. I believe it wasn't that I got taller, but that I had not shrunk. I believe that the exercise, that helped my sciatic nerve problem, stretched the vertebra at the same time as it took pressure off the disk

The irritable bowel syndrome (IBS)

Per the US News and World Report (IBS) accounts for 3.5 million doctor visits per year. (IBS) is any combination of common disturbances of the bowel/intestines, such as diarrhea and/or constipation, occurring with abdominal pain, and sometimes accompanied by physical stress. The affected body parts are the alimentary canal extension from the pyloric (opening of the stomach) to the anus. The key body process involved is the digestive process. The digestive process is completed through absorption with water, electrolytes, and nutrients. During this process the body moves along and stores fecal wastes until they are expelled. The digestive process converts food into chemical substances that can be absorbed and assimilated. During this process the body is subjected to prolonged heat and moisture so as to disintegrate and soften the food. This writer has from time to time experienced one or more of the (IBS) symptoms. I found that I was able to eliminate my (IBS) symptoms as a result of the following: First, because I was fortunate that I did not require any drugs, not even an aspirin, that in some people may cause an adverse auto immune reaction that adversely affects the body's metabolic/digestive process. Secondly, I was able to avoid ingesting any agents and/or substances that may cause an adverse auto immune reaction. I use all natural food dressings' mayonnaise, ketchup, barbeque sauce, and curry powder. Thirdly, I practiced the oriental diet, daily, of raw fruits and vegetables. This diet provided my body with enzymes and vitamins that digested efficiently within the stomach so that putrefaction and/or fermentation does not occur, both processes, which if active, would directly contribute to the (IBS). Finally, I initiated the peristalsis process on a daily basis that removed my body waste on a daily basis that if remained within the body could contribute to (IBS). As a result of following the above procedures my body's autonomic process always acted normally. As a result when I would go to bed about 9:30 pm my body's autonomic process took over with my urinary tract muscles relaxed. If I awoke at night to urinate it was always about 12:00 pm. And upon returning to bed I was fast asleep within minutes. Prior to following the above procedures I sometimes had to get up several times within the night and had to rush to urinate along with problems getting back to sleep. Now, when I awake during the night I remain in bed getting my thoughts together before slowly getting up and going to the bathroom to urinate. I next awake about 4:30 am and lie awake in bed until about 5:00 am before getting up to have breakfast. Once again thanks to my body's autonomic process I have a bowel movement sometime between 5:00 and 6:00 AM. followed by a lesser bowel movement shortly after my big meal at lunch time. Thanks to the peristalsis process and the oriental diet my stools are always odorless, soft, light colored, and only about ½ inch thick.

Constipation

Until this writer made changes in my dietary habits I had constipation problems on an interim basis, and stomach gas on a continuing basis. Once I changed my dietary habits I not only did not have any constipation period, but my bowel movements are normal and are like clockwork, and I only experienced minor gas within the bowels. Prior to detailing my changes in my dietary habits I believe it is necessary to define the constipation process. Constipation results from problems with abnormal bowel movements because of problems with storage, transportation, and evacuation of feces, from the colon. While the malabsorbtion of protein impairs a proper bowel movement the correction therein is rather straightforward. One should not eat starch with the protein in red meat since in most cases the protein is not metabolized and becomes toxic and affects the body's elimination process. However, the other key factor is more complicated and it involves the body's absorption of fiber. Fiber is the structural part of plants and plant products that consist of carbohydrates as in celluse (an inert carbohydrate), and pectin (an amorphous colloidal carbohydrate that occurs in fruits especially apples), and when eaten stimulates the peristalsis in the intestines (results in a progressive wave of contractions and relaxations of a tubular muscular system, especially the alimentary canal by which the contents are forced through the system. My diet habit changes consisted of nothing but raw fruits and vegetables, with all skins removed. I also had oatmeal and cornflakes on a daily basis. I also never ate starch, with the protein in red meat, at the same time. I found that during all meals, especially when eating raw foods, I must chew my food completely or it is constipation for sure.

Calf muscle cramps

I was taking my daily walk at a large indoor mall when I felt severe, painful, cramps in my calf muscles. I had to stop walking and had to sit down. At that time, walking directly behind me was a women security guard with the mall. I turned to her and exclaimed how painful my cramps were and that I had never experienced any thing like it in my lifetime. She informed me that she had read and/or heard that this cramping problem may be caused by the failure of the person to squarely plant their foot, when they are walking, running, and etc:. Ironically I had purposefully begun walking only on the balls of my feet thinking that this would helpdevelop my calf muscles. In particular, I was accelerating this action while going up stairs. On a daily bases I always climbed two sets of stairs at my condo. Immediately upon placing my feet squarely on the surface, particularly when going up the stairs I no longer experienced any more calf muscle cramps.

Rhinitis

Rhinitis is caused by the inflammation of the nose. This results in swelling, weeping, and redness, in the nose, which in turn results in sneezing, runny nose, postnasal drainage, and nasal congestion. Rhinitis has symptoms that are similar to both an allergic reaction and/or an adverse autoimmune reaction. Possibly the key to this problem, among some people, is a genetic problem from a hormone. I cite this example after noting the experience of some pregnant women. Some women experience rhinitis during pregnancy with the nose swelling, similar to the uterus swelling. The rhinitis increases in it's severity as the pregnancy progresses, however, after delivery the rhinitis condition automatically ends. The only suggestion that this writer can give to the reader is that they do not take any medications for this condition. Allow for the condition to self destruct. Particularly, the reader should be able to distinguish between a cold, an allergy, and/or an adverse auto immune reaction and act accordingly based on information supplied within this book.

Auricularis and associated factors

Auricularis is caused by a lack of the enzyme lactase (genetic defect). This results in a failure to catalyze lactose. As a result, there will be a build up of excess lactic acid within the body. This causes the body to develop A metabolic acidosis disease (caused by the interference with the intermediating metabolism or from the production of lactic acidosis). (caused by excessive lactic acid in the blood). The lactic acid is the end product of glycolysis. It is produced during muscle contractions as a product of anaerobic glucose metabolism. Glycolysis is formed from the catabolism of carbohydrates. Glucose is a sugar that occurs in many fruits, animal tissue, and fluids. Also, it is called starch syrup since it is obtained from the incomplete hydrolysis of starch. Glucosin is a compound that is highly toxin and is derived from a reaction to glucose with ammonia. At the same time the kidney may fail to secrete sufficient ammonia (NH4). This in turn could cause ammonaysis (wherein an ammonia group (NH2) replaces the water H2O).** As a result, ammonification takes place, and in this case, an aspergillum type fungus is produced. The net result of all of the above is the formation of the auricularis disease (a fungus covering the external parts of the ear). Also, the breath contains fungus fumes.

Associated factors Merck Def. Aspergillosis is an infectious disease of the lungs with an occasionl spread to the blood stream causes by various species of aspergillus. Otomycosis is a fungus infection of the external ear. Medical Dict. Def. Asparagine is a non essential amino acid found in many proteins in the body. It is called non-essential since only the body can make it. It acts as a drug that promotes the release of urine, it also is an excitatory neurotransmitter in the central nervous system. Aspergillosis is an infection caused by the fungus aspergillus that usually affects the ears but is capable of infecting any organ. This condition is uncommon and not easily discovered. It may also cause inflammatory granulomatous lesions on the skin, ear, or in the nasal sinus, lungs and sometimes

in the bones. Nurses Drug Manual Asparaginase (antineoplastic agent) drug is isolated from escberichia neoplastic cells and are unable to synthesize sufficient asparagines, an amino acid, to meet their metabolic needs.
This writer noticed this condition within my urine.

Note: acrylamide is a vinyl monomer that forms when a naturally occurring amino acid, called asparagines, is treated to high temps. (130 F). It is used in organic synthesis & may be toxic & carcinogenic. It may be found in French fries, potato chips, & high carbo foods.

Maple syrup urine disease

It is caused by the failure to inherit an enzyme that breaks down the amino acids that includes valine, leucine, & isoleocine! A person with this disease has a maple syrup odor in the urine! Naturally, if a person ingests any of these amino acids, per se, it will compound the problem. Amino acids are organic compounds necessary to form peptides (a molecule chain of two or more amino acids) a piece of protein, and proteins. Digestion releases the individual amino acids from the food. These essential amino acids valine (required for growth in infants and for nitrogen (N) balance in adults) leucine (essential for growth in infant and (N) balance in adults. Obtained by converting protein during the digestive process) isoleucines (required for growth in infants, (N) balance in adults) comes from the diet!Nitrogen (N) is an element that is 78% of the atmosphere, a part of proteins, and a part of most physical substances. Within a 24-hour period the (N) released by a healthy person in the urine, feces, and sweat together with the (N) kept within the skin and hair equals the (N) taken in from food and/or drink means the body is within (N) balance. The process of protein use explains the (N) balance. Most of the body's (N) is blended into proteins! Positive (N) balance is when the intake of (N) products for making tissues is greater than the (N) released. When more (N) is released than is taken in it will cause the waste and/or destruction of tissue.

Actinomycosis

Actinomycosis is a chronic bacterial disease. It is a long term medical problem that causes deep lumpy holes with thin, gravy, pus. It is often seen among patients who live in the country. It is caused by the actinobacillus bacterium that normally lives in the body's bowel and/or mouth. It is possible to inhale this bacterium. It is difficult to treat because of its dense tissue location. Other parts of the body may be affected by this bacterium. At times it is hard to diagnose since the symptoms are similar to other diseases. A former occupant of the White House developed this disease while in the White house. It is possible that the polluted White House may have housed this bacterium. At the present time the only way to prevent this disease is to maintain good dental hygiene.

Macular degeneration

MD is the leading cause of blindness in both the young and the old. Usually, one in ten people over the age of 65 develop MD. MD is a disease that destroys the macula, a tiny portion of the light sensitive retina, tissue lining the back of the eye. While the macular is only about the size of a pencil eraser it is very necessary for sight. MD occurs in two forms, the dry type that rarely leads to blindness, and the wet type which will lead to blindness, if not treated. In the wet form MD, an abnormal number of blood vessels begin rapidly growing at the back of the eye behind the retina. These cells contain large amounts of lipofuscins. It is believed that these lipfuscins are a product of the oxidative damage to the cells. The photoreceptor cells are especially affected by the above, since they use a great deal of oxygen, and are constantly bathed in light, which contributes to oxidation. This writer found that it is the failure of the proper and timeliness of the oxidation process that is the primary cause of MD. The process is complicated, since it involves the removal of electrons from an atom or a molecule. The reverse process is called a reduction reaction. Every oxidation reaction has a corresponding reduction reaction. Both reactions are influenced by the nature and strength of the bonding agents, along with the pressure and the temperature, which in turn determines the rate of the reaction. When an article appeared on MD, in a leading magazine, by a leading eye research institute, I made contact with them. Much to my surprise I received a reply from the Director of Public Affairs who wrote "I spoke with Dr. D. and she says you are right when you point out that lipofuscin build up is not the initial cause of retinal damage—the first level of damage is indeed due to oxidation". "However patients who are at risk for MD already exhibits such damage and higher than normal levels of lipofuscin, and all the evidence suggests that this substance may be the cause of the cell death that characterizes the disease". "In response to your other query, lipofuscin contains some fats, but is not itself purely saturated fat". I hate to sound like a broken record but among some people the possible prevention goes back to the diet. One must eat a diet high in fruits and vegetables. These fruits and vegetables should be raw and or not over cooked in order to preserve the vitamins and enzymes. Also, certain people must eliminate, so called, inactive substances, within food, drink, and medications, such as artificial flavoring and coloring and preservatives, since the metallic content may cause problems within the oxidation process.

ATRIAL FIBRILLATION

On more than one occasion this writer has been diagnosed with so called atrial fibrillation. Based on limited data I was unable to confirm the findings of the medical establishment. Finally, on my own I obtained data from Google and the Medical Encyclopedia that provided insight into my problem. I found that my irregular heart beat was cause by a genetically, malfunctioning mitral heart valve. I also found the reason for my long standing enlarged heart. In some people a malfunctioning of the mitral heart valve causes an enlarged heart. The latest data indicated that the mal functioning mitral heart vale may be corrected by surgery. The surgery involves taking out some extra valve tissue, and reducing the size of the ring. However, it was recommended that unless one has problems with repeated valve infections they should refrain from any surgery. Since I never had any valve infections I by passed surgery.

CAUSE AND PREVENTION OF THE FAILURE OF VACCINES

During my fact finding, involving the quality of our health care, I developed data on ingested pollutants. An article in the media caught my attention when it told about a NH. National Guardsman, who served in the Gulf war, who became sick, from what was called the gulf war syndrome. I found that many of his symptoms, outlined in the article, were similar to this writer's symptoms from accidentally ingesting polyurethane that contained as one component, isocyanine which was a component of Germany's poison gas during World War II. As a result of the above, I made contact with the Guardsman, mentioned in the article, looking for a possible connection with ingested pollutants and the so-called Gulf War syndrome. When I asked him about any pollutants that he may have come in contact with I thought I was on the right tract as a result of his reply. His duties required him to be with his motor vehicle at all times. Since this include at night, and it was cold at night, he had the heater on all night. Naturally I jumped to the conclusion that the GWS was related to ingested pollutants. However, shortly thereafter another article appeared in the media that caught my attention. The article was titled "Mother asking state to probe bad reaction to child vaccine". In the article the Mother provided examples of the adverse reactions that her son experienced from the DPT vaccine. Since many of the adverse reactions, experienced by Ryan, were similar to those experienced by the guardsman I re-contacted the guardsman and asked him if he had received any medications etc:. He indicated that he had received a vaccine and an anti nerve gas pill. In retrospect, the vaccine was an anthrax vaccine. Since the state of Mass. made their own DPT vaccine, and since the GWS affected many Guardsmen from Mass., I went to the Mass. Governors office to attempt to obtain data on the DPT and anthrax vaccines. When I showed an aide to the Governor a copy of the media article, involving Ryan, I was surprised at his response. He informed me that I should see Senator K. where they have information on the problems with the pertussis part of the DPT vaccine. I found out at Senator K's office that there were long standing problems with the pertussis vaccine. I also found out that Senator K was helping to compensate some families that had children who were adversely affected by the pertussis vaccine. I then went to the Mass. Public Health Dept. office where they did not want to talk to me. However, I did find out that there were many lawsuits as a result of medical problems associated with the pertussis vaccine. In fact an article in the media indicated that if Mass. Extended the statue of limitations, for claims relative to the P vaccine, it would overwhelm the system. In an attempt to learn more about the anthrax vaccine I made contact with the anthrax vaccine manufacture in the state of Michigan. I found that Michigan had made the anthrax vaccine to inoculate the animals to protect the animal handlers. Since it was obvious, that there were problems with manufacturing the anthrax vaccine, including deaths at the plant in Michigan, I went back to Senator K"s office. Once they found out all the information that I had collected on the pertussis and anthrax vaccines they could not escort me out the door fast enough. On the way out I indicated to the senator's staff that I was going across the street to the US. Attorney's office. When I arrived at the US. attorney's office, it was obvious they were expecting me and could not escort me out the door fast enough.

At this point reports began to surface linking the GWS and the anthrax vaccine. In one article it said that the anthrax vaccine is suspect in the GWS. The Associated Press reported that the safety of the anthrax vaccine given the troops was being challenged. Also, the AP reported that it was believed that the brain damage, found among some sick Gulf War Vets, could be traced to the anthrax vaccine.

At this point I began to collect documented data on vaccines but more specifically the DPT and the anthrax vaccines. In one report doubts were raised about vaccinations. It reported that that some if not all, vaccinations may presently do more harm than good. It cited all the adverse reactions to some vaccines. It was indicated that the DPT vaccine was a suspect in sudden infant death syndrome. A UCLA study published in the 1980's showed one major seizure for each 875 children immunized with the DPT vaccine. This represented a reaction rate more than ten times as great as the study generally cited by pediatricians.

I believe that the problems with the anthrax and DPT vaccines involve two processes, with one of the processes involving the possible cause and prevention of the failure of vaccines. The first process and the reason for the similarity of problems with both the DPT and the anthrax vaccines is that both vaccines are of the whole bacillus type bacteria. Most vaccines use only part of the bacteria and they are not usually of the bacillus type bacteria. Unfortunately the whole bacillus bacterinum lends itself to the endospore/endotoxin process.

Endospore/endotoxic process

(**Source**—The biology problem solver, research and education association)

Some bacteria have the capacity to transform themselves into highly resistant cells called endospores. In the process, know as sporulation, bacteria forms these intracellular spores in order to survive adverse conditions, such as extremely dry, hot, or cold environments. Each small endospore develops within a vegetative cell. Each vegetative cell is the form in which these bacteria grow and reproduce. Each endospore contains DNA in addition to essential materials derived from the vegetative cell. All bacterial spores contain dipicolinic acid, a substance not found in the vegetative form. It is believed that a complex of calcium ion, dipicolinic acid, and peptidoglycan, forms the cortex or outer layer of the endospore. This layer or coat helps the spore to resist the destructive effects of both physical and chemical agents. The dipicolinic acid/calcium complex may play a role in resuming metabolism during germination. The spore is generally oval or spherical in shape and smaller than the bacterial cell. Once the endospore is mature, the remainder of the vegetative cell may shrink and disintegrate. When the spores are transferred to an environment favorable for growth, they germinate and break out of the spore wall, and the germinating spore develops into a new vegetative cell. The endospore is incapable of growth or multiplication. This in turn results in the development of an endotoxin, a polysacharin, which in combination with a lipid is released from the cell walls of gram negative bacteria producing a toxic effect (fever, shock). Endospore formation is neither a kind of reproduction nor a means of multiplication, since only one spore is formed per bacterial cell. During spore formation, a single endospore is present within the bacterium. The remaining portion of the vegetative cell dies off, while the endospore remains to later germinate into a new vegetative cell. This new vegetative cell is identical to the old one because it contains the same DNA. Spores only represent a dormant phase during the life of the bacterial cell. This phase is initiated by adverse environmental conditions. Endospore definition endo, is inside the cell and/or body while spore is a bacterial form that is resistant to heat, drying, and chemicals and may change back into an acting form of the bacterium. Diseases caused by the spore forming bacteria are the anthrax, botulism, gas gangrene, tetanus, and pertussis.

Bacteria in the genera Bacillus and Clostridium are partially characterized by their ability to form endospores. Spores of the bacillus anthracic, the bacteria causing anthrax can germinate 30 years after they are formed. The bacillus type bacteria are found within both the anthrax and the pertussis, (whooping cough,) vaccines.

Bacterial growth can usually be determined by measuring cell number, cell mass, or cell activity. Growth refers to the increase in size of the individual organism. In bacteria it is the number of cells increased over the initial quantity used to start the culture (called the inoculum). Some species of bacteria require only a day to reach their maximum population size, while others require a longer period of incubation. Growth can usually be determined by measuring cell number, cell mass, or cell activity. ENDOTOXIN, the polysaccharin that is combined with a lipid is released from the cell wall of the gram negative bacteria producing toxic effects causing fever, and shock. POLYSACCHARIN a group of complex carbohydrates, such as starch, that decomposes by hydrolysis into a large monosaccride unit. LIPID a group of organic compounds consisting of fats and other substances of similar properties. They are insoluble in water but soluble in alcohol and other organic solvents. They are stored in the body cells as a energy reserve. A poison is released when the bacteria dies.

One look at the above and there should be no doubt in anyone's mind that, not only do the vaccines fail to metabolize, but they develop medical problems as a result of the endospore/endotoxic process. In this process, a wall is formed around the bacteria, usually from metals, such as those in preservatives, which results in an unmetabolized vaccine. At some point the bacteria breaks through the metal wall, resulting in a toxic reaction.

CAUSE AND PREVENTION OF ADVERSE REACTIONS TO DRUGS

Background

Within this section I have attempted to provide the reader with documented data that will allow them to protect themselves against adverse reactions to drugs.

The reader should address problems with medications similar to the less serious problems with ingested pollutants. The reader must address problems with medications with consideration given that every body is different as to how they may react to a specific drug and/or quantity of a drug, along with the accumulation of all drugs. However, what is most important is that the reader must recognize that the so called inactive agents and/or substances in the drug itself may be viewed by the body as a foreign agent, and may cause the body to have an adverse auto immune reaction.

This writer found that the body's adverse reactions to medications were usually not as a result of the basic drug chemistry. The adverse reactions to drugs were primarily caused by the wrong drug and/or the wrong dosage and/or a combination of both. The wrong drug and or the wrong dosage could be affected by a person's age, gender, along with a person's height to weight ratio. All of the above, including the drug itself, may be affected by the type and/or quantity of the so called inactive agents and/or ingredients, such as colorants and preservatives, that are added to the drugs. These agents and/or substances may not only alter the drug's chemistry, but they may cause an adverse autoimmune reaction that may cause the drug to fail to metabolize. The above may be compounded by a medication overdose, particularly among the elderly.

Prior to providing specific details on various medication problems I believe the reader should be aware of several factors that are the precursors to many medication problems. The first key factor is the inability of the FDA to properly monitor the development, testing, and the reporting, of adverse reactions to new

91

drugs. I believe an article in the media says it all.. The article was titled Report faults FDA drug safety unit. The article indicated that the FDA office, responsible for policing the safety of prescriptions drugs, is under funded, understaffed, and lacks a clear and effective process for deciding whether, and how, to act, when it determines a drug is unsafe. When the departing secretary of health and human services, Tommy Thompson, endorsed the creation of a new independent agency, to monitor prescription drugs, after they are on the market, he helped save the proposal from becoming buried under the pharmaceutical industry's opposition. The Senate should press Thompson's proposed successor, Mike Leavitt, on this issue at his confirmation hearings. Still, creation of such an office is just one of many steps needed to protect the public from the dangers, such as the cardiovascular problems linked to the long-term use of two popular pain killers. Monitoring is now done by an office, within the FDA, that lacks sufficient funding. Its staffers also know that any decision they make, to demand tougher label warnings or even suspend drugs, is an implied criticism of their colleagues, who approved them. Whether a new, strengthened, drug review, office is set up inside or outside of the FDA, adequate funding from Congress will be crucial. Over the years, the review office has seen its staffing actually decrease even as more and more drugs come on the market. This is as a result of Congress's stinginess, and a 1992 agreement with drug companies that shifted more government and industry money into speeding approvals of new drugs for diseases like AIDS and cancer. By all means, life-saving drugs should not be kept off the market because the FDA's new drugs office lacks staffers. However, even that office, which is well funded, should reexamine procedures that let a non-life-saving drug like Vioxx on the market after safety testing that was not rigorous enough to reveal its long term effects on the cardiovascular system.

The slowness, with which the FDA addressed the issues, involving antidepressant drugs, demonstrates another problem. Studies that pointed to problems with these drugs were often suppressed by the drug companies that sponsored them. More-positive results, of course, quickly found their way to the pages of the leading medical journals, a chief source of information for doctors, and into the hands of the drug companies' sales people. Another major source of doctors' information between drug makers and patients are phalanxes of professionals who should ensure the safety and effectiveness of medications: researchers, FDA reviewers, medical journal editors, and doctors. All of them depend on impartial, fully transparent information to do their jobs right. In any changes Congress makes, that goal should be foremost. In another media article that ties in with the above "HARVARD RESEARCHERS SAYS FDA APPROVAL RULES TOO

LAX" speaks for itself. In this article it stressed that US regulators approve drugs without knowing enough about their risks. The Harvard researcher said that the FDA rules too often focus on irrelevant measures, such as how a drug compares to a placebo. The article went on to say that it is more important to weigh risks and benefits against drugs already in use. Any Americans gullible enough to believe that the drug industry can be trusted to fully report on what clinical trials it is sponsoring or what results were found must be sorely disappointed by recent developments. A government survey determined that three of the largest drug companies have effectively reneged on their pledges to list trials in a federal database. A report in the Times reveals that this intransigence also extends to a voluntary industry database. It looks as if demands from researchers and the medical profession for full access to clinical trial data will continue to be frustrated. Companies already provide the data to the Food and Drug Administration, which is required to keep much of it confidential. A public listing of trials is important to prevent drug makers from hiding results that reflect badly on their drugs while publishing only the results that make their drugs look good. By law, the companies are supposed to register important trials within a government Web site. Most manufacturers are complying, but the three big obfuscators are often getting around the requirement by not naming the drugs they are testing, instead using phrases like "an investigational drug". It was also reported, that meager contribution appears to satisfy the weak guidelines set by the industry, but it offers a sorry contrast with the record of one other leading drug company who appears to have been quite scrupulous in listing its current trials within the government site and has posted the results of hundreds of completed clinical trials on the industry site. Surely if one big company can make its trials transparent, other drug makers can do the same. A coalition of medical editors has just stiffened its announcement that leading journals will soon refuse to publish the results of any clinical trial that has not complied with tough international standards for transparency. That should apply useful pressure to recalcitrant companies, but the best hammer would be federal legislation to compel all companies to provide critical information when a trial is begun and full results when a trial is completed, with stiff penalties for noncompliance.

Key drug actions affecting drug metabolism

Adverse interactions between drugs There are instances in which the therapeutic or adverse effects of drugs are modified by the administration of a 2nd drug and/or agent. With each prescription, the possibility for interaction between drugs should be considered. One drug may potentate a 2nd drug thereby producing adverse effects, or may nullify its usual therapeutic, actions. Therapeutic effects are antagonized by any agent that interferes with the delivery of a drug to its site of action in the body. This may occur if the absorption of the drug is impaired, if the rate of its metabolism is enhanced, or if the transport mechanism which carries the drug to its cellular site of action is blocked. Conversely, inhibition of the drug's metabolism or competitive displacement of a drug that is tightly bound to plasma protein will enhance the delivery of the drug to its site of action, thereby increasing both therapeutic and adverse effects. In addition to these interactions resulting from changing the amount of drug available to the target organs, there are some interactions that result from alteration of the response of the target cells them selves.

Interference with the delivery of a drug at the drug site Interference with absorption, chelating: Some drugs (e.g., the tetracycline's) form strong chelating complexes with metallic ions, which render the drug unavailable for absorption thus, antacids, containing magnesium and aluminum, are given together with a tetracycline, formation of chelates in the intestinal tract will prevent absorption of the antibiotic. Ion exchange resins the ion exchange resin cholestyramine, is used to bind bile acids in the intestinal tract, thereby preventing their reabsorption. This resin also binds a number of drugs, impairing their absorption. Cholestyraramine prevents the absorption of orally administered thyroxine and liothyronine (triiodotbyronine) in man. In experimental animals this resin impairs absorption of other drugs, including digitoxin, aspirin, secobarbital, and phenylbutazone. Because the full range of drugs sequestered in the intestinal tract, by cholestyraznimine, it has not been explored, it is, suggested that any drug should be given at least 1 hr before cholestyraznimine.

Delivery of an excessive quantity of drug to the drug site This action may cause the inhibition of the metabolism of a drug as well as increase the duration and magnitude of its action. Certain drugs are bound strongly to plasma proteins and in this physical state are pharmacologically inactive. This reversible binding is primarily to the albumin fraction of plasma protein. A number of drugs compete for common binding sites, and this is a basis for drug interaction. When displaced from plasma proteins by another drug, an agent becomes available in the unbound and pharmacologically active form, and its effect is intensified. Added to the above was that it was found that 20% of new drugs recommend dosages are too high.

Wrong prescription More than 7.9 million elderly receive the wrong prescriptions. Compounding all of the above was the report by the AMA on the actions of common drugs on women versus men. It was found that the common aspirin works better on men than on women to prevent heart attacks, while it protects women better than men in the prevention of strokes. Also, there is the failure on the part of the MSE to properly address the part that ingested pollutants play in the proper metabolism of drugs. Meanwhile, the doctor is presented with a problem when he or she has to become familiar with so many new drugs, sometimes as many as sixty in one week. If the doctor took the time to become completely familiar with all the new drugs she or he would not have time to practice medicine. As a result, when the patient comes in to the doctor's office and asks for the latest drug on the market for their medical problem the doctor willingly gives it to them with no questions asked and the patient is out the door. Also, the doctor usually is only criticized if they don't medicate at the right dosage so it is usually medication for sure at the maximum dosage. The AARP reported that in a study of 354 drugs introduced in the US from 1980 to 1999 20 percent of recommended dosages were too high. In part, as a result of the above, when the patient has an adverse reaction to the initial drug a second drug is given for this reaction without eliminating the first drug. At times this could mean drug after drug prescribed to address adverse reaction after adverse reaction. While anyone may be affected by the above approach, to solving medical problems, it appears that senior citizens are more susceptible to medication errors.

FDA doctor's response The FDA doctor's response to this writer's two inquiries says it all. I first asked the FDA doctor who was responsible for up dating drugs on their interaction with other drugs and ingested pollutants? His response was "that is a good question". I then asked the FDA doctor if I should be concerned about preservatives and their adverse reaction on the body's autoimmune process. His response was "I always check every package and if it has preservatives in it I never buy it". He caught me off guard so I forgot to ask him what he does about medications that usually have preservatives in them.

A few medication problems affecting the pending death of health care

Hormones and breast cancer The media article indicated that the medical scientificestablishment (MSE) found that women taking hormones, particularly estrogen (E) on along term basis, 10 years, for problems associated with menopause have been contracting breast cancer. Once the women, in the study group, stopped taking estrogen the overall breast cancer rate dropped by 7% between 2002 and 2003, with a 12% decrease in breast cancer among women ages 50 to 69. I believe that the reason for the higher decrease among women 50 to 69 is that as we age our metabolic process, including metabolizing medications, is less effective thereby compounding the problems with medications. The key documented data within the physicians' desk reference are as follows: Under warnings (E) have been reported to increase the risk of endometrial carcinoma in post menopausal women. (E) should not be taken by pregnant women. While the majority of studies have not shown an increase risk of breast cancer in women who have used (E) replacement therapy, some have reported a moderately increased risk (relative risks of 1.3-2.0) in those taking higher doses or those taking lower doses for prolonged periods of time, especially in excess of 10 years. In all my years of collecting documented data on drugs I have never encountered as many inactive ingredients in any other drugs that I encountered in (E). Inactive ingredients listed were acacia, calcium carbonate, carnauba wax, carboxymethylcellulose sodium, citric acid, colloidalsilocon dioxide, diacetylated monoglyceride, gelatin, anhydrouslactose, magnesium stearate, methylparaben, microcrystalline celluse, pharmaceutical glaze, povidone, propylparaben, shellac, sodium benzoate, sodium bicarbonate, sorbic acid, sucrose, corn starch, talc, titanium dioxide, and tribasic calcium phosphate. Also, in addition to the above they were the colorant coatings that relate to the drug dosage. For example, for the 0.3 mg tablet there is the fd & c blue #1 lake colorant. Also, added to the above, that I have never seen in any other drug, is the label imprinting ink containing black iron oxide, fd&c blue #2 lake, fd&c red #40 lake and fd&c yellow #6 lake. For the 2.5 mg tablet the imprinting ink contains soya lecithin, dimethyl polysiloxane, pharmaceutical shellac, and titanium dioxide. There are at least six, so called, inactive ingredients listed in the above that this writer has not had an allergic reaction to, but an autoimmune reaction to. The cause of the problem between the (E) and breast cancer is centered on the body's reaction to the accumulation, compounding and/or synergetics of the in gestation of the (E) with all its, so called, inactive ingredients, and/or in combination with the in gestation of other drugs with similar inactive ingredients. Naturally, the higher the dosage, the higher the inactive ingredients, in the drug. Also, as we age we develop more fat body cells than lean body cells and any accumulation of drugs and their inactive ingredients may collect within the body's fat cells compounding the problem. As a result of the above, the body's adverse auto immune process is activated. In this process, a type of antibody, the cytolysin, is released and it attacks the red blood cells of the breast causing damage and/or destruction resulting in breast cancer. Recently, The University of Texas M.D Anderson Cancer Center reported that from 2002 to 2003 there was the single largest drop in cases of breast cancer in one year. They attributed this drop to the decrease in the use of hormone therapy. To provide the patient with an (E) that will serve its purpose without causing other medical problems I recommend that as many so called inactive ingredients, particularly colorants and preservatives, be eliminated. I believe the implementation of my medical patent PERFECT PRESCRIPTION PACKAGE #530579, as outlined in the manuscript section SUGGESTIONS AND PRO-POSALS FOR A HEALTHY LIFE; will address any concerns about the removal of colorants, indicating dosage, and the preservatives, that maintain the colorant.

The article in the media indicated that a leading medical writer for a paper died of an overdose at a leading cancer research and treatment center. This writer found that in her treatment two drugs were involved. One drug was to suppress the body's immune system in order to allow for the cancer drug to work effectively. The other drug was the cancer drug. Unfortunately, at times, it is difficult to properly suppress the body's immune process so there is a tendency to over apply the cancer drug hoping to overcome the body's immune process. Unfortunately this often ends up with a drug overdose..

There was the 90 year old women who was taking heavy doses of the anti hypotension drugs Lorazepam, Reserpine, and Lisinopril. The Lisinopril was given to her to replace the Reserpine because she was experiencing severe adverse reaction. Reserpine is a hydrochlorothiazide that is a diuretic and an anti hypertensive drug. These combinations of drugs are not recommended for initial therapy for hypertension. The Doctor's continued to prescribe both the Lisinopril and Reserpine for this woman. As a result of the adverse reactions, to these drugs, the woman was forced to wear a diaper at all times and when at home had to sit along side the bathroom that was on the second floor.

There was the woman in her sixties that went to a women doctor at a leading NH. hospital with an apparent vaginal infection. During this visit the doctor reported that this woman had a heavy discharge and a fishy odor from the vagina. The woman was not informed of this condition by the doctor the women learned of this from her medical report. The woman did not have any of these symptoms the symptoms were right out of the drug manual for anyone having a problem with gardnerella bacteria. The doctor prescribed 4 capsules of metronidazole to be taken at the same time. The manufacture recommends this drug for trichomonas only. On the second visit to the doctor, the doctor prescribed 2 500 mg of metronidazole per day for 7 days. Per the manufacture the dosage for trichomonas is 250 mg. for ten days but taken by both the woman and her husband. The woman requested that the doctor take a pap smear. The woman had a severe adverse reaction to the medication so she stopped taking this drug. The genital culture report indicated that this woman had normal vaginal flora. The doctor did not report this to the woman she had to find out by reviewing her medical records. Also, during this period the doctor never instructed the woman to stop taking the drug. This writer believes that the prescribing of the wrong drug at the very high dosage caused an autoimmune reaction. This reaction caused swollen biathlon's glands in the vagina. As a result the swollen glands blocked the normal lubrication of these glands which led to a dry vagina with irritation. The irritation affects the bacillus bacteria balance in the vagina opening it to possible infections. Finally, in a study of 800 women in Scandinavia those women that took the drug M for other than T had high cervical cancer rates. In an attempt to prevent anyone else from having similar problems the doctor was requested to file a report with the FDA she refused. The drug manufacture was contacted and was given the details of the doctor prescribing the wrong drug at the wrong dosage. The drug manufacture was asked to file a report but not only refused but said "we don't care what the doctor uses our drug for or at what dosage".

There was the two year old girl that went to the pediatrician with pressure within the ears from inflammation. The doctor prescribed 500mg. of amoxicillin (A) per day. This writer suggested to the mother and father that they not give this high dosage of amoxicillin to their daughter. This writer indicated that based on my experience as a child, with severe ear infections, their daughter could not possibly have a severe ear infection calling for 500 mg. of A since she experienced no pain. Upon checking with the manufacturer of A I found that the manufacture did not recommend giving this drug to anyone two years or younger, and the maximum dosage for children was 45mg. In retrospect this was not a true ear infection but an autoimmune reaction causing the inflammation of the inner ear canals. If this girl had taken this drug, particularly at the maximum dosage, she could have damaged her hearing fibers resulting in a hearing loss. This is what happened to Pres. Clinton, causing a hearing loss.

This writer as a result of a personal experience had problems with two drugs digoxin and diltizem used for atrial fibrillation and the drug coumadin used as a blood thinner. Up until the point that I became involved with these drugs I was fortunate in not requiring any drugs not even an aspirin. All along my pulse readings were 68 with the average 60 to 100. My blood pressure readings were systolic 112 with the average 140 or less and diastolic 85 with the average 85 or less. My problems started when I went to my PCP complaining of breathing problems especially while lying down. I did not have any breathing problems while exercising. I also never had any chest pains and/or heart palpations. My PCP checked and found that I had an enlarged heart. To the best of my knowledge I have had an enlarged heart since I was a young man. My PCP recommended that I take two drugs digoxin and diltizem since he detected some atrial fibrillation problems. Despite taking these drugs my breathing problems continued and I attempted to get my PCP to reconsider my treatment but he refused. I then went out of state to an ER where they found that I had a nonmalignant bleeding tumor in the stomach. It was the bleeding that causes a loss of oxygen hence the breathing problems. The hospital found that my hematocrit was only 19.% when it should have been 43%. Based on this writer's findings the medical profession followed the normal practice of never stopping a drug, particularly if you were not the person who prescribed the drug in the first place. As a result they continued to give me the same two drugs for atrial fibrillation. When my fibrillation problem did not change they gave me a larger dosage. Once again not only was there no change in my condition I developed an autoimmune reaction to the increased dosage. In retrospect this was from the increase in the amount of preservative in the two drugs. Prior to this point I would have an adverse autoimmune reaction to not only a preservative per se, but to the quantity of the preservative. At the same time they attempted to give me an antacid drug that the medical manual indicated that if taken with digitalis it would affect the absorption of that drug. Fortunately, I pretended to take the medications but threw them away. After the operation to remove the tumor they attempted to give me a pain pill even though I did not have any pain. I believe that the CVS print out on the drugs diltazem and digoxin along with the information in Delmar's nurses drug reference manual says it all. In the CVS print out diltazem is listed as a calcium channel blocker" digoxin promotes "the intracellular concentration of calcium" "The displacement of the calcium and/or potassium by digoxin caused heart fibrillation problems (irregular) in some people". In the CVS drug interaction section "tell your doctor of all prescriptions you may use especially digoxin". In the Delmar's nurse's drug reference under digoxin drug inter action "diltiazem increases digoxin serum levels. Under diltizem drug interaction "digoxin serum levels increases are possible". Is it possible that after reading the above that it is logical to conclude that these two drugs, that are used for heart fibrillation problems, are probably the cause for the 450,000, yearly, deaths from heart rhythm problems. At this writer's suggestion I replaced the above two drugs with the drug coumadin, a blood thinner, and/or anticoagulative. Per the manufacture, in patients with non rheumatic atrial fibrillation coumadin significantly reduces the risk of systemic thromboembolism inducing strokes. It was found that the reduction of thromboembolism or prevention of strokes was the same for either the moderately high dosage with 2.0 to 4.5 INR readings or the low dosage with a 1.4 to 3.0 INR (international normalizing ratio) readings. Basically, it inhibits the synthesis of vitamin K.. Also, it was found that in the elderly, 60 years or older, a patient required less coumadin to produce a therapeutic levels of anticoagulative. This writer believes that this is as a result of the failure to metabolize the coumadin causing a build up of the drug. Elimination of coumadin is almost entirely by metabolism. Coumadin is responsible for more adverse drug reactions than any other drug. The pharmacy print out on coumadin warned the user not to take any aspirin while taking this drug. My PCP became upset with me when she wanted me to increase my dosage of coumadin in order to raise my INR ratio to above 2.0. My INR ratio at the time was 1.4 which the manufacture says is acceptable. Also, when earlier I attempted to increase the dosage I had an adverse reaction to the preservative in the drug so I was afraid of an overdose. My PCP would not listen to me and when I went for a refill at the pharmacy at the lower dosage of coumadin I was informed by the pharmacist that my PCP was no longer my PCP. At this point I just stopped taking the drug period and so far I have had no adverse effects.

President Clinton, while in office was taking a so called diet pill/heart burn drug that had to be pulled from the market because of over 38 associated deaths. Imagine, we are not talking about a strong anti biotic and/or a blood pressure pill, but a simple diet pill. The media reported that a space shuttle astronaut nearly died from an allergic reaction to an experimental drug during a NASA medical experiment.

A recent study found that medication errors are plaguing nursing homes. It found that one out of every 10 nursing home residents suffers a medication related injury. In another study it found that more than 7.9 million elderly received incorrect prescriptions. In a recent study it was found that over medication, of the elderly, particularly of those living alone, had reached epidemic proportions and has become a national health problem.

In a study by a leading University it found that 20% of recommended dosages of new drugs are often too high.

In a recent study it was found that adverse reactions to common drugs put 700,000 people into emergency rooms. Also, the study indicated that this figure was probably conservative since adverse drug reactions are often misdiagnosed.

A drug disaster by a **leading drug company** If anyone would have told this writer, before I began my fact finding, on our health care problems, that one of the biggest and best drug company in the world would have to recall a drug, because of it's serious adverse reactions, that had been successful on the market for over a decade I would have thought that they were out of their mind. This drug, that sold extensively within the US., and outside the US., was a genetically engineered version of the human protein! This drug had freed millions of patients with cancer and kidney disease from their reliance on blood transfusions. The first paragraph of the media article of 11-27-02 says it all "! It's the worst fear of every drug maker when a drug that has been on the market for more than a decade and has brought in billions in revenues suddenly begins causing a potentially deadly condition in the very patients it is meant to help"! The article further stated that the drug in question "was causing the body's natural defenses to go hay wire and attack its own red-blood cells "how dangerous the immune response to their drug can be and how poorly understood they remain "! Per usual, since the medical scientific establishment MSE does not understand the body's adverse autoimmune reaction the MSE made no comment. One key example of how badly the process was misunderstood was the comment in the article that "the immune system sometimes produces neutralizing antibodies to fend off what it views as foreign invaders"! The person who made this statement doesn't have a clue as to how the autoimmune process functions. In the article it mentioned that one of the reactions was an attack on the red blood cells. This is a perfect example of the autoimmune process since it involves the protein cytotoxin, which acts like an antibody, and attacks the cells of the various parts of the body. Another key statement was that this company believed that the problems "are linked to the manufacturing changes made shortly before the problems began". Once again it points to this writer's data on the causes of the body's adverse auto immune reaction. I found that the worst statement made by this fine company, in the article, was "existing lab tests don't always forecast how manufacturing changes will affect a drug"! This writer without any training and/or education, in this field, could pin point the problem without any lab tests! The sad part of the above fiasco was that this fine drug assisted many people. Unfortunately, the problems that this fine Company experienced in their attempts to make this drug came down to their failure to recognize that the problem involves the body's autoimmune process! Ironically, the Company's feeling that their problem stemmed from manufacturing changes was right on the money! Any changes in the colorants used and/or the types of preservatives and/or a combination of both could have triggered an autoimmune reaction causing the drug to fail to metabolize!

The not so reliable aspirin During my many months of collecting documented data on the plight of our health care these findings on the aspirin were a real shocker. The cause of the problems with the absorption failures of aspirin, as outline in the media articles, ties in with this writer's findings. The problems with the aspirin are the same problems that were experienced by other drugs. The articles in the media, as indicated, provided information on the lack of benefits for some people who take the baby aspirin. "ASPIRIN,: UP to 40% of PEOPLE GET NO HEART BENEFITS FROM IT" More than 20 million Americans regularly take aspirin, but new studies say between 5% and 40% aren't getting benefits because they're "aspirin resistant." Aspirin's well-know benefits: it helps to prevent blood clots and, thus, heart attacks and strokes. It also is cheaper and has fewer side effects than prescription anticoagulants. Your doctor can tell if you are resistant to aspirins by ordering a simple "platelet aggregation test" that checks how your blood is clotting. This can be part of your regular check-up. The article in the media went on to say "WHEN YOUR ASPIRIN'S A BUST". "Over 50? At risk for heart disease? Taking a daily aspirin is a great idea for most people who fit this description, but some patients receive no benefits-possibly because they're taking the wrong pill. Coated aspirin can reduce stomach irritation, but the coating may prevent the drug from being absorbed, say doctors at Dublin's Royal College of Surgeons. They gave 75 people low-dose aspirin every day for two weeks, then measured blood samples, coated aspirin was absorbed at only two-thirds the rate of uncoated aspirin. The results need to be confirmed, says a member of the American Heart Association, but he's already advising some of his patients to switch to uncoated aspirins. This writer found that people are called "aspirin resistant" because they have had an autoimmune reaction. This autoimmune reaction to the so called inactive agents, in the baby aspirin, causes the blockage and/or reduction in the enzymes necessary to metabolize the 81mg baby aspirin. Also, it is possible that the coating on the baby aspirin could lead to a chelating reaction that could cause the aspirin to fail to be absorbed. For example: one look at the definition of the aspirin ingredients indicates that it contains the active chemical salicylic which is derived from salicylic acid that is prepared from salicin or phenol and since salicylic is an active agent it was not listed on the package. Listed on the package were the so called inactive ingredients D&C Red #27, Aluminum Lake and FD&C Red #40 Aluminum Lake. Many people have adverse reactions to these agents. The 325mg aspirin does not have any of these so called inactive agents that are contained within the baby aspirin, and as a result there is no adverse autoimmune reaction to the 325mg aspirin. If this writer was to take an aspirin I would take one quarter of the 325mg aspirin.

Pain pill problems The AP reported on 12-20-06 that the federal Health Officials say that the pain pill warnings must be tougher. It went on to say that Americans, who take the popular over the counter pain pills, face potentially serious side effects. These pills include aspirins, ibuprofens, and acetaminophens. The article went on to say that, in regard to an overdose of acetaminophen*, it could cause serious liver damage. In regard to aspirins and ibuprofens and other non steroidal anti inflammatory drugs there is a risk of gastric intestinal bleeding and kidney damage, even in those patients that take the correct dosage. Doctors say that the problems are compounded when the patient takes two or more medications, say one for pain, and another for the flu symptoms, knowing that they both contain acetaminophen.**

The federal Health officials will require the drug companies to put warnings on the pain pill packages. The report stated that the feds. attempted to have these warnings placed on the pain pill packages before, but the drug companies rejected it. As noted, when the body's adverse autoimmune process is triggered by the so called inactive ingredients, within the pill, it may cause the pill not to metabolize and that may result in a drug overdose. Also, it is important to note that the pills chemical reaction is anti inflammatory; while the body's adverse auto immune chemical process is inflammatory.

*It is an amide of acetic acid and p-aminophenol, anon prescription drug having analgesic and antipyretic effects similar to aspirin, but only with weak anti inflammatory effects.

**Why would the person have this information, when some of the information was just revealed, by this AP article?

The process for getting a drug approved in the U.S. is rigorous, but it isn't designed to detect every possible risk. That would require studies so large, and so long that few new medicines would ever hit the market.

Problems with the FDA After a drug or device is allowed on the market, the FDA and the drug's maker are supposed to watch for evidence of new risks among its users. The FDA oversees a database that gets reports of about 280,000 incidents a year of potential adverse drug reactions. About 90% of those reports come from drug makers, who are required to disclose them; doctors and other medical personnel aren't required to participate in this report process. By some estimates, FDA's database may reflect only a few of such incidents. The reports are sometimes of limited value, since it is hard to pinpoint for sure that a drug is the cause of a problem. Some researchers have argued that the reporting database needs to be supplemented by more active studies to search for and confirm safety problems of drugs already in broad use. For instance, a 1998 editorial in JAMA called for a new "office of drug safety with the authority, independence, funds, and legal mandate" to more actively track problems. Once a drug is approved, the FDA doesn't have the authority to order a company to do a safety study, but it has indirect leverage because if it has strong enough evidence it can force labeling changes or take a drug off the market. As part of the approval process, the FDA can also sometimes require that so called phase four studies be done later, after the drug goes on the market. A FDA report in March said that through Sept. 30,

2003, the agency had 1,338 outstanding post-marketing commitments for drugs, with 65% of the studies not yet initiated. The FDA has said it is monitoring the compliance with such commitments. A few years ago, drug companies pulled a number of medicines off the market or severely restricted their use because of dangerous side effects. Among them were a diabetes drug that could cause liver failure, an anti cholesterol medication that was tied to higher rates of muscle problems than its competitors, and a diet-drug. The FDA has defended its decisions, generally saying it relied on the evidence available at the time, and had to balance the benefits against the risks. The Senate Finance Committee and the House Energy and Commerce Committee made their requests for the GAO study of how the FDA responds to safety concerns after both panels investigated FDA officials' initial decision not to allow a staffer to publicly present his conclusion that antidepressants could be linked to suicidal tendencies in young people. The FDA said it thought that conclusion was premature when the staffer reached it in February. The FDA later confirmed the finding through further analysis unveiled in August and plans to put a warning on the drugs' labels. An FDA spokeswoman says the agency's reviewers and its safety analysts agree "the vast majority of the time" and have "a lot of collaborating back and forth." The FDA said they are moving to improve how it finds and responds to risks from medical products, including trying to do better data-mining of adverse events and using electronic filing to process reports. The agency is examining health-care provider data, he said. It also hopes to stimulate new scientific research to improve the design of clinical trials of drug safety and promote research on pharmacogenetics, which may help to identify which people will react badly to drugs. In the past few years, the FDA has also been more active in imposing conditions on use, when a drug is approved to limit its potential risks

Points for the reader to consider involving drugs

I hope up to this point I have provided sufficient documented data to the readers, regarding medications, to alert them to protect themselves. However, if the reader is not convinced by my documented data they should recall the statement made by a doctor who is the head of clinical trials at a leading drug company. His comment was "that consumers would have no new drugs if all safety risks had to be eliminated first". Also, the reader should consider the statement by various drug makers on a common adverse reaction to their new drugs. They claim that of all the adverse reactions that they reference, to their drugs, the most common is the dry mouth. It appears that they not only accept this as a matter of fact but give the impression that it is insignificant. Unfortunately the dry mouth is not insignificant, but it may be serious for some people. A dry mouth indicates no saliva. No saliva indicates swollen saliva glands from the body's adverse autoimmune reaction to what the body perceives as an ingested foreign agent including the medication itself. No saliva means no digestive enzymes in the mouth to assist in the body's digestive process. A loss of these enzymes means not only improper digestion per se but the possible failure of the body to properly digest the medication itself which could cause a drug overdose.

Finally, the U.S. Agency for Healthcare Research and Quality recommends that the readers exercise the ultimate in self help by asking your Doctor and/or Pharmacist the following questions: what is the name of the medicine? Is it ok to substitute a less expensive generic medicine for the name brand and will it achieve the same effect? What is the dose of the medicine? Are there any foods, drinks, other medicines, or activities that I should avoid while taking this medicine? What are the possible side effects and what should I do if they occur? How many refills of this prescription can I get? What should I do if I miss a dose? Is there written information I can take home? In the latter case the patient should ask the Pharmacist for the drug manufactures print out on the drug which contains most of all of the above data.

Specific data on the cause and prevention of adverse drug reactions

Anemia drug I believe that the problems associated with the cause and prevention of the adverse reactions to anemia drugs provides the basis for addressing the cause and prevention of adverse reactions to all drugs. As a result of deaths, in clinical studies, the FDA has issued its most severe warning possible for drugs used to treat anemia, in kidney disease patients, and cancer patients, under going chemotherapy. The major problem with the original anemia drug came about when the inventor created the multiple dosage anemia drug. The so called preservatives that he put into the multidosage formulation were not preservatives in the truest sense, but anti bacterial agents. Treatment beyond recommended limits increases the risk of deaths from heart attacks and strokes in kidney patients, and of tumor growth and deaths in cancer patients. The FDA advised doctors to give the minimum dosages, and indicated that the drug should not be used to improve the quality of life, for cancer patients. A doctor, at a leading cancer center, said "these drugs have been somewhat over used". "There has been, I think, for patients, and to some extent health providers, to attribute more fatigue to anemia than deserves to be attributed". A clinical trial of Procrit, called CHOIR, was cut sort because of higher rates of deaths, from heart attacks, and strokes, in kidney patients, receiving higher doses than those recommended by the FDA. In another report of a study of Aranesp, in cancer patients, not undergoing chemotherapy, they found a higher percentage of deaths.

I believe that the Doctors dictionary says it all about anemia, and this ties in with this writer's findings. The adverse reaction to anemia drugs ties in with the body's adverse autoimmune reaction to an ingested foreign agent and/or substance such as preservatives. The drug fails to properly metabolize, resulting in an overdose. Amgen, the anemia manufacture, recognizes this problem since they have a drug, less preservatives. Anemia is a reduction below normal in the number of erythrocytes in the hemoglobin. The autoimmune hemolytic involves a large group of anemia's; involving auto bodies, and usually involves sequestration of sensitized erthrocytes by the spleen

A leading drug company had their patent expire on the anemia drug epogen. Another leading drug company attempted to make this drug, but had to recall their version because of serious side effects. The original drug company replaced the epogen with a better drug called aranesp. The drug company that was unsuccessful, in making the drug epogen, obtained a license, from Amgen, to sell epogen under the name procrit. Naturally, one has to raise the question why would anyone want any of the anemia drugs but aranesp. In 2006 the sales were epogen, original form, 2.5 billion, procrit, identical to epogen, 3.1 billion, and aranesp, a better epogen, 4.1 billion. These revenues were mostly from Medicare reimbursements. I don't know how the US public will understand the above, particularly the epogen/procrit arrangement.

First of all, the adverse reaction to the anti anemia drugs is caused by the body's adverse auto immune reaction. BAAR. However, prior to providing details on this process it is important for the reader to understand what might trigger this reaction. The so called preservatives and additions, such as polysorbate 80 contained within the multi dosage anti anemia drug composition are the agents and/or substances that trigger the BAAR. Normally, preservatives within food, drink, and medications, are there to prevent oxidation, the spoiling of food and drink, and the loss of the colorant, in medications, that denotes the dosage of a drug. The so called preservatives placed within the composition of the multi-dosage anti anemia drug is not there to prevent oxidation, but to prevent bacteria from entering into the composition, which could adversely affect the drug itself, and/or directly adversely affect the recipient of the drug. In other words the so called preservatives protect the drug from anaerobic decomposition of organic matter by a bacteria and/or fungus. Using Mr. Strickland's, the inventor of the anemia drug, own words these so called preservatives are used as an antimicrobial agent. Most important through out the definitions of these so called preservatives the key words used in identifying their function are germicide, bacteriostatic, fungi static & sterilizing agents. No where is the word preservative used in identifying their functions, since that is not their function..

Most important, while we reference the so called preservatives in reference to the body's adverse auto immune process there are other agents and/or substances, that in conjunction with the so called preservatives, may cause problems with the body's auto immune process at the same time as the so called preservatives are causing adverse reactions. For an example of how complicated the process is one only has to review the inability of a leading drug company to make an anemia drug that had been on the market for ten years. See data on drug disaster by leading drug company.

The failure to properly address problems with the anti anemia drugs that involves $9.7 billion is one of the precursors to the death of health care in the US.. Compounding the problem is the fact that we have members of the medical scientific establishment that have doubts that there are any serious problems with these drugs. The FDA drug safety podcasts issued by Pat Clarke of the FDA's center for drug evaluation and research, should dispel any doubts about the problems with these drugs. However despite this report Dr. Pazdur FDA stated that "No evidence high doses of anemia drugs can be fatal". Also, there are conflicting statements among people who were directly involved in the problems with the anemia drug Procrit. Dr. Singh, Brigham and Women's Hospital, who supervised the Choir trials of J&J, s drug Procrit stated, "I was surprised by negative reaction". Meanwhile, J&J's Craig Tendler VP. Orth Biotech stated, "We remain confident on the safety and efficiency of Procrit when used according to the label".

First, we must eliminate the so called preservatives and most of the other additions. In other words, any agent and/or substance, that its prime function is antimicrobial. Naturally, since there is still a danger that a bacteria will enter into the process, steps must be taken to prevent this from happening. While, since my knowledge of the overall drug chemistry is very poor, I believe that there are two points in the process that may be prone for the intrusion of bacteria. The first and most important is the albumin human blood serum. The second point, within the process, that lends itself for the intrusion of bacteria, is at the point on the skin of the injection of the drug. In addition to addressing the above problems, I believe that a study should be under taken of the effect that lymphaocytes and/or monokines have on the body's immunological process, during the absorption of the anti anemia drug.

AVANDIA DRUG

For another example of problems with the adverse reaction to drugs I would like to cite the example of the Avandia drug. The media reported that the world's best selling diabetes drug last year will carry US. regulators strongest warning on the risk of heart attacks. The FDA's action fell short of restrictions on Avandia that were put in place in Canada and Europe in recent weeks. Canada withdrew approval and Europe would only use it in selected groups of patients.

The problems with the Avandia drug are in line with most adverse reactions to drugs. Per the manufactures print out the Avandia drug contains the following so called inactive ingredients, hypromellose 2910, lactose monohydrate, magnesium sterate, microcry stalline, microcrstalline cellulose, polyethylene plycol 3000, sodium starch glycolate, titanium dioxide, triacetin, and one or more of the following synthetic red and yellow iron oxides and talc.

Any of the above so called inactive ingredients per se and/or compounded by similar ingredients in food and or other medications ingested at the same time as ingesting the Avandia drug may trigger the body's auto immune process.

On a personal basis if had I ingested the Avandia drug, the so called inactive agents in the drug, lactose monohydrate, magnesium sterate, titanium dioxide and the synthetic red and yellow iron oxide would have triggered my body's adverse auto immune process (see autoimmune definition in the chapter on EFFECTS OF BODY PROCESSES)

Based on my personal experience the adverse auto immune reaction would cause the improper metabolism of the Avandia drug that in effect creates a build up of the Avandia drug, resulting in a drug overdose. It is this drug overdose, in some people, that causes medical problems including heart attacks

SUGGESTIONS AND PROPOSALS FOR A HEALTHY LIFE

Upon the reader developing a medical problem they should contact Google for the basic data on that medical problem. In place of the implementation of the MUST patent, see below, prior to the Doctor prescribing any drugs for the patient they should contact Google for all up to date data on that drug. Also the patient should provide the Doctor with the names of all the drugs that they are taking at the present time. Using this information, the Doctor will contact Google and obtain all adverse reactions to the drugs per se. Also Google will provide data on any adverse reactions of the drugs as a result of the inter action of any of the drugs..

Keeping in mind that Japan is the healthiest nation in the world, adopt their diet and lifestyle. Their diet consists of very little red meat, but if eaten it is always eaten without starch. It is composed of skinless, raw fruit and vegetables, particularly leafy vegetables, on a daily basis. The diet allows for the enzymes and the vitamins in the raw food to digest very efficiently, within the stomach, so that the calories are burned efficiently. One of the key enzymes is called cellulose. It is an inert carbohydrate. This enzyme breaks down the fiber of whole grains, vegetables, fruits, and nuts that normally resist digestion in the gastrointestinal tract. As a result, a person doesn't experience the gastric ills of putrefaction (an action that causes matter to rot and/or decompose, particularly proteins and organic matter, with the production of foul smelling compounds such as hydrogen sulfate, ammonia, and mercaptans), and fermentation, as in yeast enzymes, molds, and certain bacteria, (an action that decomposes carbohydrates that in turn form acetic, butyric, and/or lactic acids). The Japanese feel strongly that their ingesting of ample amounts of fiber has contributed to their good health. The fibers involved consists of carbohydrates such as cellulose or pectin and in particular amorphous colloidal carbohydrate that occur in fruits especially apples. While in Japan I found that they had a diet of leafy vegetables twice per day. I have found that when I follow the above diet, including the leafy vegetables twice per day, I have a normal daily bowel movement upon awaking at 5:00 am. The Japanese food is always warm, never hot, so as to not lose any enzymes and/or vitamins by overheating. Unlike China, who has at least 1700 fast food establishments, Japan has no fast food establishments thereby eliminating fried foods, with their trans fat.

On a daily basis assist the body's autonomic process, in particular the peristalsis process, (creates waves of contractions and/or relaxations of the tubular muscular system, especially the alimentary tract), by which the body's solid waste contents are forced through the system. This process is activated by ingesting carbohydrates, such as celluse and/or pectin, and in particular the amorphous colloidal carbohydrates found in fruits, especially apples.

By following the Japanese diet, along with promoting the body's peristalsis process, I believe that the digestive tract and the colon/rectal tract have no long term bacteria.

Adopt the life style of the Japanese, which is fewer automobiles, more public transportation, and more walking than Americans. This diet and lifestyle has resulted in no obesity in Japan.

If you experienced any of these body reactions on a continued bases: dry itchy skin, itchy eyes, dry throat, pressure within the inner ear, frequent trips to urinate, particularly at night, balance problems, particularly when getting up from a sitting and/or reclining position, they are caused by an adverse auto immune reaction to something that you have ingested.

Avoid ingesting adverse autoimmune triggers and preservatives as defined in the section on the EFFECTS OF INGESTED POLLUTANTS.

Avoid the accumulation, compounding, and/or synergetic, of so called inactive agents within food, drink, and/or drugs since this may cause an adverse auto immune reaction.

Consume fresh fruits on an empty stomach, since most fruits pass directly into the small intestine.

Avoid eating eggs and red meat at the same time since they contain two major proteins and the pancreas has trouble releasing the two different enzymes for proper digestion.

Avoid ingesting large amounts of wheat (gluten) since it may affect the normal liver function.

Vasopressins in food and drink such as cheese, wine, chocolate, grapes, and nuts may restrict blood vessels reducing the flow of oxygen.

Alcohol slows the burning of body fat in some people by as much as 31%.

While we are all aware that we must chew our food properly and eat and drink slowly I don't believe that the average person realizes that chewing food properly takes a lot of time. If one is successful in chewing food properly there is no solid food particles left prior to ingesting the food.

Separate starch and red meat by at least 12 hours since the pancreas can't produce both enzymes required to process them both at the same time. The chemical process involved is very complicated. Acid and alkaline juices are secreted simultaneously in response to the incoming protein and starch. As a result the protein and the starch promptly neutralize one another leaving a weak watery solution in the stomach that digests neither the protein and/or the starch properly. As a result the protein putrefies and the starch ferments as a result of the constant presence of bacteria in the digestive tract. The blood stream picks up the toxins from the putrefied, fermented mess sending the toxins throughout the body attacking the red blood cells. Even birds eat worms at one time and seeds at another time.

Avoid burnt red meat since the protein in the meat will not metabolize.

Avoid eating any very hot and/or very cold foods since metabolic and/or degradation rates may be affected.

The body requires some fat for overall body metabolism and assimilation. The ratio of fiber to fat is usually 75% to 25%. This ratio is very critical and if not maintained the body is unable to propel the bulk throughout the body, thereby, not assisting the body's waste elimination process.

Eat nothing that won't spoil and/or rot if not eaten, but eat it before it spoils and/or rots.

Don't ingest any large amounts of food and/or drink just prior to exercising and/or just after exercising, and just prior to going to sleep. The body's chemistry during the exercise and/or sleep cycles doesn't allow for the proper metabolism of the agents and/or substances within the food and/or drink.

We should be so lucky, the best solid dog food has no hydrogenation of oil, no artificial flavors and/or coloring, and no preservatives.

Since the present approach to resolving medical problems, by the medical establishment, is always after the fact by cure and treatment it makes sense that the reader, friends, colleagues, and other interested parties should propose establishing a panel, of lay people and medical professionals, to address the cause and prevention of medical problems. Unlike the present time, where large financial medical research grants are awarded up front, the very large medical grants should only be made upon the discovery of the cause and prevention of a medical problem.

Develop a hormone and enzyme replacement program.

That the drug companies accept the AMA's proposal for a total drug try out disclosure that should include safety concerns once the drug is approved.

Eliminate the use of off label drugs.

The FDA should alter the monitoring system on new drugs. The time between the discovery of a problem with a new drug and the voluntary and/or regulatory removal of the drug from the market should be measured in months not in years as under the present system

The FDA should establish new drug labels with clear and concise information on the chemical reactions involved along with the ingredients. In order for the FDA to implement the above they should become independent of the pharmaceutical industry. Congress should make the FDA an independent agency with adequate staffing and funds to maintain the surveillance of the safety of drugs from their inception to their after marketing performance. Back Senator Kennedy in his proposal to revamp the FDA.

Within your state promote the plan implemented by Pennsylvania. Pennsylvania found that two million Americans contracted infections after being admitted to the hospital and 90,000 died. They decided to attempt to inform the public by publishing a booklet on all the hospitals, within their state, listing the patients that contracted infections upon entering a specific hospital. This will allow the reader to help themselves by selecting a hospital with limited problems associated with the above. Naturally, it is hoped that by going public, with this data, the hospitals will change their ways of operating.

Suggest that the reader consider acting on the results of a recent report in the British Media. The report found that middle age whites were healthier in England than their counterparts in America. Also, it was found that the richest third of Americans had as much diabetes and heart disease as the poorest third of the English. It was found that Americans have more obesity than the English. The above was evident despite the fact that the English and Americans life styles, relative to diet, drinking, and smoking, appeared to be similar. I believe the reasons for the above is that the English use less autos for transportation and more walking and public transportation. I compared the English lifestyle to the Japanese life style and found that the Japanese do even more walking than the English and are much healthier and have no obesity period. For exercise Americans should walk several times per week.

If possible put the air conditioning and heating systems on vent prior to starting them up at the beginning of the season. This is an attempt to purge any pollutants within the ducts. Also, when running the systems always allow for the system to complete the cycle and shut off on its own. This helps to prevent any residue such as moisture within in the ducts to possibly turn into a pollutant. If after performing the above you still develop a reaction to the duct air which, some people call a cold, you should hire a professional to clean the ducts.

The AMA should adopt this writer's two proposed medical patents. These two proposed patents are "**PERFECT PRESCRIPTION PACKAGE**" or PPP #538579. and "**MEDICAL UPDATE SOFTWARE TOTAL** or MUST.

PERFECT PRESCRIPTON PACKAGE (PPP) PATENT # 530579

This patent would allow for the elimination of all artificial flavors and/or coloring along with preservatives within all medicine capsules and/or tablets.

This package consists of three parts. First, a bottom, of a plexiglas type material, about 2.5 wide, with a length to be determined by the user. This bottom will have pockets about one half inch square and three eights inch deep that will hold the medication capsules, and/or tablets. Secondly, there will be a top covering the entire bottom, of Plexiglas type material, with a lip type seal. Thirdly, there will be a sheet of wax paper type material covering the entire top. This sheet will contain the color code for the medication dosage, along with any preservative necessary to maintain the color, and will also have any imprinted information relative to the medication. This package if designed correctly will allow for the removal of one or more pockets, with the medication in it, without jeopardizing the integrity of the package.

MEDICATION UPDATE SOFTWARE TOTAL (MUST) # 530580 PATENT

This patent would prevent the misapplication and/or wrongful dosage of medications per se. Also, to identify and remove from the medications any ingested agents and/or substances that maybe adversely affect the body, causing the inhibition of any enzymes required to properly metabolize the medication. Failure to properly metabolize the medication could result in a drug overdose and/or an increase in the medication's serum levels.

A computer software program should be created with three parts that will match the correct medication and/or dosage for the patient's medical problem. Also, the same program will identify any agents and/or substances that could cause the inhibition of any enzymes required for the proper metabolizing of the medication.

PART 1 A permanent database less any data on pregnant women, nursing Mothers, children under two years old, and any person with special needs. It would include the name of all medications and their generic names and the purpose of the medication. It will also include data on the correct medication at the correct dosage for the person's age, gender, height, and weight. The data base will include the medications ingredients, pharmacology, and pharmacokinetics data. It will also include any medication overdose data along with any reported adverse reactions. All of the above will be updated periodically.

PART II The input to the data base will include the patient's mental and/or physical symptoms along with any lab reports etc: related to the patient's medical problem. Included will be the patient's medical history and body profile. Also, include will be all data on all drugs including non prescription drugs that the patient is taking, along with any enzymes and/or supplements presently taken by the patient.

PART III The output from the above will consist of a written report with the patient's and the Doctor's signature. This report will include the name of the drug and dosage recommended, including the generic drug name and the correct dosage recommended. It will include the drugs chemical ingredients, including the inactive ingredients along with any applicable drug pharmacology and/or pharmacokinetics data. Also listed will be all the drugs and their dosage presently being taken by the patient along with any supplements herbs etc: presently being taken by the patient.

The comments by a Doctor at the FDA, and an epidemiologist says it all! When this writer indicated, to a doctor at the FDA. about my concerns over the adverse effects on a persons health from preservatives within food and drink, and my concerns over who was responsible for updating data on the adverse interactions between drugs responded "I always check every package and if it has preservatives in it I never buy it" and as to drug interaction updates "that is a good question"! An epidemiologist reported that he spent two years talking with his colleagues and two hospital visits before finding out that his medical problems were caused by a common food colorant! The FDA Doctor should have looked at himself in the mirror for the possible answers!. While the FDA. sets up requirements for the allowable amount of preservatives within a particular substance they have no requirements for the total all allowable amounts and/or their strengths of all preservatives within a given substance! In regard to any adverse reactions to the body, from drugs, the FDA. requires only voluntary reporting of any adverse reactions! So, unless there is any obvious problems, with disabilities and/or deaths, the FDA. will not issue a recall! In some cases the adverse drug reaction is reported by the drug company as if it is insignificant but it isn't! For example, one of the common side effects to many drugs is a dry mouth! However, a dry mouth means no saliva and no saliva means no ptyalin enzymes for metabolizing starch and no mucin enzymes for the protection of the mouth from abrasions! In some cases where no direct deaths are involved a new drug is developed to replace the drug causing the adverse reactions without removing the older drug! Unfortunately, the patient continues to take the old drug along with the new drug! Also, with some drugs not only is the serious adverse effect not immediately noticeable but it is hard to pin point the exact drug involved! As a result, there are 450,000 deaths, per year, from heart rhythm drugs with the FDA. unable to address the problem despite the obvious cause!

Within the patent Perfect prescription package (PPP) problems with any adverse reactions to preservatives and/or colorants within drugs are addressed by their elimination!

Within the patent Medication update software total (MUST) any problems, involving the adverse reactions between drugs etc., along with the daily up dating of any adverse reactions, involving all drugs, are properly addressed as they relate to a particular body profile! However, more important, in addition to providing the above information the MUST patent properly addresses the requirement to address any problems involving auto immune reactions and their triggers!

The implementation of the **Must patent** will prevent a recent serious event from happening in the future. A doctor was being sued for his failure to warn his patient that the drug he prescribed for him could cause serious sleepiness. As a result, the patient fell asleep, while driving, and ran off the road killing a pedestrian on the side of the road. The Must patent provides the patient with a print out of all the side effects and etc along with any side effects associated with any other drugs that the patient may be taking.

Finally, this writer had two catch 22 episodes as a result of my involvement with the body's adverse auto immune process. When this writer had my bout with the auto immune disease Sjogren Syndrome I experienced every adverse auto immune reaction in the book. In particular, I had swollen saliva glands with a loss of saliva with its digestive enzymes, and a very dry mouth. As noted, this condition was a precursor to Alzheimer's disease. Also, at the same time I had a swollen bladder reducing the capacity of the bladder, forcing me to get up several times during the night to rush to the bathroom to urinate. Today, as a result of my diet, and avoiding ingesting pollutants, I not only do not have a single adverse auto immune reaction I find myself drooling profusely, at night, while in bed. Also, I find myself awakening only about twice during the night and finding myself lying awake awhile before realizing I need to urinate, prior to casually going to the bathroom to urinate

Meanwhile, while the above takes place, despite the change in time, my body continues to function like a finely tuned timepiece. I go to bed about 9:30 and go right off to sleep. As a result of my muscles relaxing I awake at about 11:30 and casually go to the bathroom to urinate. I then awake at about 2:00 and casually go to the bathroom to urinate. Upon returning to bed I go back to sleep. I next partially awake, about 4:00, and fully awake about 5:00. At times I do take a one hour nap during the afternoon. I am never on this schedule to urinate during the day; it is only because my body's muscles are relaxed, during the sleep cycle that I am on that schedule at night.

978-0-595-47704-3
0-595-47704-6